T0229325

Advanced Imaging in Gastroenterology

Guest Editor

RALF KIESSLICH, MD, PhD

GASTROENTEROLOGY CLINICS OF NORTH AMERICA

www.gastro.theclinics.com

December 2010 • Volume 39 • Number 4

SAUNDERS an imprint of ELSEVIER, Inc.

W.B. SAUNDERS COMPANY

A Division of Elsevier Inc.

Elsevier Inc. • 1600 John F. Kennedy Blvd., Suite 1800 • Philadelphia, Pennsylvania 19103-2899

http://www.theclinics.com

GASTROENTEROLOGY CLINICS OF NORTH AMERICA Volume 39, Number 4
December 2010 ISSN 0889-8553, ISBN-13: 978-1-4377-2525-4

Editor: Kerry Holland
Developmental Editor: Jessica Demetriou

© **2010 Elsevier Inc. All rights reserved.**

This journal and the individual contributions contained in it are protected under copyright by Elsevier, and the following terms and conditions apply to their use:

Photocopying

Single photocopies of single articles may be made for personal use as allowed by national copyright laws. Permission of the Publisher and payment of a fee is required for all other photocopying, including multiple or systematic copying, copying for advertising or promotional purposes, resale, and all forms of document delivery. Special rates are available for educational institutions that wish to make photocopies for non-profit educational classroom use. For information on how to seek permission visit www.elsevier.com/permissions or call: (+44) 1865 843830 (UK)/ (+1) 215 239 3804 (USA).

Derivative Works

Subscribers may reproduce tables of contents or prepare lists of articles including abstracts for internal circulation within their institutions. Permission of the Publisher is required for resale or distribution outside the institution. Permission of the Publisher is required for all other derivative works, including compilations and translations (please consult www.elsevier.com/permissions).

Electronic Storage or Usage

Permission of the Publisher is required to store or use electronically any material contained in this journal, including any article or part of an article (please consult www.elsevier.com/permissions). Except as outlined above, no part of this publication may be reproduced, stored in a retrieval system or transmitted in any form or by any means, electronic, mechanical, photocopying, recording or otherwise, without prior written permission of the Publisher.

Notice

No responsibility is assumed by the Publisher for any injury and/or damage to persons or property as a matter of products liability, negligence or otherwise, or from any use or operation of any methods, products, instructions or ideas contained in the material herein. Because of rapid advances in the medical sciences, in particular, independent verification of diagnoses and drug dosages should be made. Although all advertising material is expected to conform to ethical (medical) standards, inclusion in this publication does not constitute a guarantee or endorsement of the quality or value of such product or of the claims made of it by its manufacturer.

Gastroenterology Clinics of North America (ISSN 0889-8553) is published quarterly by Elsevier Inc., 360 Park Avenue South, New York, NY 10010-1710. Months of issue are March, June, September, and December. Business and Editorial Offices: 1600 John F. Kennedy Blvd., Suite 1800, Philadelphia, PA 19103-2899. Customer Service Office: 6277 Sea Harbor Drive, Orlando, FL 32887-4800. Periodicals postage paid at New York, NY and additional mailing offices. Subscription prices are $282.00 per year (US individuals), $142.00 per year (US students), $458.00 per year (US institutions), $310.00 per year (Canadian individuals), $558.00 per year (Canadian institutions), $392.00 per year (international individuals), $195.00 per year (international students), and $558.00 per year (international institutions). Foreign air speed delivery is included in all *Clinics* subscription prices. All prices are subject to change without notice. **POSTMASTER**: Send address changes to *Gastroenterology Clinics of North America*, Elsevier Health Sciences Division, Subscription Customer Service, 3251 Riverport Lane, Maryland Heights, MO 63043. Telephone: 1-800-654-2452 (U.S. and Canada); 314-447-8871 (outside U.S. and Canada). Fax: 314-447-8029. E-mail: journalscustomerservice-usa@elsevier.com (for print support); journalsonlinesupport-usa@elsevier.com (for online support).

Reprints. For copies of 100 or more, of articles in this publication, please contact the Commercial Reprints Department, Elsevier Inc., 360 Part Avenue South, New York, New York 10010-1710. Tel. (212) 633-3813, Fax: (212) 462-1935, E-mail: reprints@elsevier.com.

Gastroenterology Clinics of North America is also published in Italian by Il Pensiero Scientifico Editore, Rome, Italy; and in Portuguese by Interlivros Edicoes Ltda., Rua Commandante Coelho 1085, 21250 Cordovil, Rio de Janeiro, Brazil.

Gastroenterology Clinics of North America is covered in *MEDLINE/PubMed (Index Medicus)*, *Excerpta Medica*, *Current Contents/Clinical Medicine*, *Science Citation Index*, *ISI/BIOMED*, and *BIOSIS*.

Printed and bound by CPI Group (UK) Ltd, Croydon, CR0 4YY

Transferred to Digital Print 2011

Contributors

GUEST EDITOR

RALF KIESSLICH, MD, PhD
Professor of Medicine, I Med Klinik, Universitätsmedizin Mainz, Mainz, Germany

AUTHORS

SHARMILA ANANDASABAPATHY, MD
Associate Professor of Medicine, Gastroenterology, The Henry D. Janowitz Division
of Gastroenterology, Mount Sinai School of Medicine, New York, New York

RAJA ATREYA, MD
Professor of Medicine, Medical Clinic I, University of Erlangen-Nuremberg,
Erlangen, Germany

JACQUES J.G.H.M. BERGMAN, MD, PhD
Associate Professor of Medicine, Department of Gastroenterology and Hepatology,
Academic Medical Center, Amsterdam, The Netherlands

MARCIA IRENE CANTO, MD, MHS
Associate Professor of Medicine and Oncology, Division of Gastroenterology and
Hepatology, Department of Medicine, Johns Hopkins University School of Medicine,
Baltimore, Maryland

CHRISTIAN FOTTNER, MD
Department of Endocrinology and Metabolism, I Medical Clinic, University of Mainz,
Mainz, Germany

MARC GIOVANNINI, MD, PH
Head of Endoscopic Unit, Paoli-Calmettes Institute, Marseilles, France

LORENZA ALVAREZ HERRERO, MD
Department of Gastroenterology and Hepatology, Sint Antonius Hospital, Nieuwegein;
Department of Gastroenterology and Hepatology, Academic Medical Center, Amsterdam,
The Netherlands

ARTHUR HOFFMAN, MD
I Med Clinic, Johannes Gutenberg University of Mainz, Mainz, Germany

MOSTAFA IBRAHIM, MD
Gastroenterology and Hepatology Department, Theodor Bilharz Research Institute, Cairo,
Egypt

MITSURU KAISE, MD, PhD
Director, Department of Gastroenterology, Toranomon Hospital, Minatoku, Tokyo, Japan

MASAYUKI KATO, MD, PhD
Department of Endoscopy, The Jikei University School of Medicine, Minato-ku, Tokyo, Japan

RALF KIESSLICH, MD, PhD
Professor of Medicine, I Med Klinik, Universitätsmedizin Mainz, Mainz, Germany

CHANG-QING LI, MD, PhD
Department of Gastroenterology, Shandong University Qilu Hospital, Jinan, China

YAN-QING LI, MD, PhD
Director and Professor, Department of Gastroenterology, Shandong University Qilu Hospital, Jinan, China

ANDREA MAY, MD, PhD
Department of Internal Medicine II, HSK Wiesbaden, Wiesbaden, Germany

MATTHIAS MIEDERER, MD
Department of Nuclear Medicine, University of Mainz, Mainz, Germany

MARKUS F. NEURATH, MD
Professor of Medicine and Director, Medical Clinic I, University of Erlangen-Nuremberg, Erlangen, Germany

HORST NEUHAUS, MD
Professor of Medicine and Chief, Department of Internal Medicine, Evangelisches Krankenhaus, Düsseldorf, Germany

DON C. ROCKEY, MD
Professor and Chief, Division of Digestive and Liver Diseases, University of Texas Southwestern Medical Center, Dallas, Texas

JENNY SAUK, MD
Instructor of Medicine, Gastroenterology, The Henry D. Janowitz Division of Gastroenterology, Mount Sinai School of Medicine, New York, New York

HISAO TAJIRI, MD, PhD
Professor, Department of Gastroenterology and Hepatology, The Jikei University, Minato-ku, Tokyo, Japan

GRISCHA TERHEGGEN, MD
Doctor of Medicine, Department of Internal Medicine, Evangelisches Krankenhaus, Düsseldorf, Germany

ANDRÉ VAN GOSSUM, MD, PhD
Department of Hepato-Gastroenterology, Erasme Hospital, Free University of Brussels, Brussels, Belgium

MAXIMILIAN J. WALDNER, MD
Resident, Medical Clinic I, University of Erlangen-Nuremberg, Erlangen, Germany

JEROME D. WAYE, MD
Director of Endoscopic Education, Mount Sinai Hospital; President, World Endoscopy Organization (WEO/OMED); Clinical Professor of Medicine, Mount Sinai Medical Center, New York, New York

MATTHIAS M. WEBER, MD
Professor, Department of Endocrinology and Metabolism, I Medical Clinic, University of Mainz, Mainz, Germany

BAS L.A.M. WEUSTEN, MD, PhD
Department of Gastroenterology and Hepatology, Sint Antonius Hospital, Nieuwegein; Department of Gastroenterology and Hepatology, Academic Medical Center, Amsterdam, The Netherlands

Contents

This review discusses the application of 2 novel imaging techniques in Barrett's esophagus: autofluorescence imaging and narrow band imaging (NBI). Autofluorescence as well as NBI may help to direct endoscopic therapy for early neoplasia in Barrett's esophagus; their value in daily practice, however, seems to be limited and needs further evaluation.

Endomicroscopy is a remarkable technical advance in gastrointestinal mucosa imaging. In 2003, Kiesslich and colleagues described the first human use of contrast-aided confocal laser endomicroscopy (CLE) as a novel technique for in vivo microscopic imaging of the gastrointestinal mucosa. Both probe-based and endoscope-based systems have been applied to many gastrointestinal disorders, including Barrett's esophagus (BE) and associated neoplasia. Probe-based confocal laser endomicroscopy can be used in conjunction with highresolution white light endoscopy and other contrast enhancement techniques. It has proven high accuracy for prediction of high-grade neoplasia and cancer. In vivo imaging of both flat BE and mucosal lesions can influence diagnosis and thereby impact upon decision making regarding tissue sampling and endoscopic therapy. This article discusses the scientific literature related to clinical use of CLE for BE, the techniques for performing CLE in the esophagus, and the potential future directions for CLE in BE and esophageal cancer diagnosis and treatment.

Gastric cancer is the third common cancer and is the second leading cause of cancer deaths worldwide. Endoscopy is being increasingly used for gastric cancer screening because of a high detection rate. Despite promising data, the technique depends heavily on the availability of endoscopic instruments and expertise for mass screening. Furthermore, the introduction of various new endoscopic devices and techniques may enhance the value of endoscopy in efficacious cancer screening. High-definition endoscopy and image-enhanced endoscopy, including narrow band imaging, are the key modalities in advanced endoscopic imaging in gastric cancer.

In vivo histologic diagnosis of gastric intestinal metaplasia (GIM) and gastric cancer (GC) can be achieved by confocal laser endomicroscopy (CLE).

This review describes the endomicroscopic features of GIM and GC and reviews their clinical applications. Differentiation of phenotypes of GIM and GC by using CLE is also discussed.

Andrea May

Nowadays, 5 nonsurgical flexible endoscopic techniques are available for small bowel endoscopy: push enteroscopy (PE), balloon-assisted enteroscopy using 2 balloons (double-balloon enteroscopy [DBE]) or 1 balloon (single-balloon enteroscopy [SBE]), balloon-guided enteroscopy (BGE), and spiral enteroscopy (SE). PE is a cost-saving, easy, and fast procedure for the examination of the proximal jejunum, but for a deep small bowel endoscopy, the other flexible enteroscopic techniques are required. BGE does not play a considerable role in deep small bowel endoscopy. DBE is the oldest flexible enteroscopic technique. Actually, the balloon-assisted enteroscopy (BAE) techniques with one balloon (SBE) or two balloons (DBE) are the mainly used techniques. DBE has become established throughout the world for diagnostic and therapeutic examinations of the small bowel and is now used universally in clinical routine work. DBE is still regarded as the gold standard nonsurgical procedure for deep small bowel endoscopy, because it provides the highest rates of complete enteroscopy, which becomes increasingly useful. The recently introduced SE technique represents a promising method but still needs technical improvement. Larger prospective studies on SE and prospective studies comparing the 3 systems (DBE, SBE, SE) are awaited before conclusive assessments can be made.

André Van Gossum and Mostafa Ibrahim

Video capsule endoscopy (VCE) that was launched 10 years ago has become a first-line procedure for examining the small bowel, especially in the case of obscure gastrointestinal bleeding. Other major indications include Crohn disease (CD), celiac disease, and intestinal polyposis syndrome. In the case of small bowel diseases, the use of VCE must be integrated in a global diagnostic and therapeutic approach. More recently, wireless endoscopy has been adapted for examining the colon, opening up larger perspectives for colorectal cancer screening or colon examination. Technologic modifications of the second-generation colon capsule increase the sensitivity of this method for detecting polyps. Other new developments, including remote magnetic manipulation, power management, drug delivery capsule, microbiopsy capsule, and adaptation of technologies such as chromoendoscopy, are sure to enhance the capabilities of wireless endoscopy in gastrointestinal disorders.

Grischa Terheggen and Horst Neuhaus

In the evaluation of biliary diseases, cholangioscopy is considered as complementary procedure to radiographic imaging. Direct visualization of the bile duct is the premier advantage of cholangioscopy over indirect imaging techniques. However, cholangioscopy has not gained wide acceptance because of several technical limitations such as scope fragility, impaired steerability, limited irrigation, and suction capabilities, as well as the need for two experienced endoscopists. Recent innovations such as the implementation of electronic video cholangioscopes and the development of single-operator systems facilitate the procedure, and promise to increase the diagnostic and therapeutic yield of cholangioscopy.

Recent progress of the data processing applied to ultrasonographic (US) examination has made it possible to develop new software. The US workstation of the last generation thus incorporated in their center a computer allowing a precise treatment of the US image. This advancement has made it possible to work out new images such as 3-dimensional (3D) US, contrast harmonic US associated with the intravenous injection of contrast agents, and even more recently, elastography. These techniques, quite elaborate in percutaneous US at present, are to be adapted and evaluated with endoscopic US (EUS). The contribution of contrast agents of US to pancreatic EUS and then 3D EUS are successively approached in this article.

New high-resolution colonoscopes and filter technologies are allowing us to visualize more lesions and better characterize lesions within the gastrointestinal tract. In light of recent findings that flat and serrated lesions are more likely to contain invasive cancer and that even small lesions (5–10 mm) may contain advanced histology, detecting these lesions earlier with improved optical technologies may help decrease the rate of interval cancers after colonoscopy. With the limited accuracy of white-light colonoscopy (59%–84%) in distinguishing non-neoplastic lesions from neoplastic lesions, these new technologies can help us improve our abilities to risk stratify patients and determine more precise surveillance intervals.

Colonoscopy is the best imaging device currently available for the detection of lesions in the large bowel, but may be an imperfect tool against colon cancer. Because recent guidelines for colorectal cancer screening and surveillance depend on whether polyps are found on colonoscopy and on their size, the need to identify all the neoplasia in the colon has assumed greater importance. This article reviews and assesses the latest developments in colonoscopy including wide-angle optics, endoscope caps and hoods, retroflexion and the use of the third eye retroscope.

Computed tomographic (CT) colonography is a noninvasive method to evaluate the colon and has received considerable attention in the last decade as a colon-imaging tool. The technique has also been proposed as

THE CLINICS ARE NOW AVAILABLE ONLINE!

Access your subscription at:
www.theclinics.com

Preface

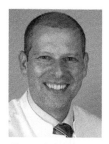

Ralf Kiesslich, MD, PhD
Guest Editor

As Guest Editor, it is my great pleasure to introduce this issue of *Gastroenterology Clinics of North America* devoted to Advanced Imaging in Gastroenterology.

Advances in imaging in gastroenterology have led to new insights and diagnostic algorithms. Patients with gastroesophageal reflux disease face an increased cancer risk. Here, new imaging modalities like narrow band imaging, endomicroscopy, and autofluorescence enable better visualization and targeted biopsies of Barrett's esophagus associated neoplasias.

Gastric cancer is still a major killer in Asian countries. Thus, it is absolutely essential to adequately screen populations at elevated cancer risk. Here, magnifying endoscopy enables visualization of the fine details of gastric cancers, which can be used for early detection, which is a prerequisite for endoscopic treatment. Endomicroscopy is able to visualize even premalignant conditions such as atrophic gastritis or intestinal metaplasia of the stomach.

The small bowel can now be fully visualized with different technologies. Capsule endoscopes can be maneuvered and can also explore the large intestine. Complete enteroscopy with endoscopes is possible with different techniques that enable endoscopic therapy in almost all regions of the human gut.

Bilopancreatic diseases have a great impact on the reduction of the quality of life of the affected patients. New imaging options like cholangioscopy and contrast-enhanced endosonography open the door for early detection of these diseases.

Colonoscopy is still standard for screening of colorectal cancer; however, colonoscopy is not perfect and can be improved with wider and retro views. Also, better optics and filter techniques can increase the detection rate and help to better understand the nature of colorectal lesions. CT colonography is almost established in the United States, whereas it is controversially discussed in other parts of the world.

Finally, personalized medicine is an upcoming trend, and molecular imaging will be the method of choice to tailor therapy with biologicals or smart molecules. Molecular imaging is already used for the detection and treatment of neuroendocrine tumors, but molecular imaging will also be a factor in endoscopy in the near future.

Gastroenterol Clin N Am 39 (2010) xiii–xiv
doi:10.1016/j.gtc.2010.09.001
0889-8553/10/$ — see front matter © 2010 Elsevier Inc. All rights reserved.

gastro.theclinics.com

The articles in this issue will broaden your knowledge about advanced imaging modalities and help you to better understand the possibilities—and limitations—of modern imaging.

I have to thank all of the authors for their extraordinary efforts, their friendship, and their scientifically outstanding contributions.

Ralf Kiesslich, MD, PhD
I Med Klinik
Universitätsmedizin Mainz
Langenbeckstr 1
55131 Mainz, Germany

E-mail address:
kiesslic@mail.uni-mainz.de

Autofluorescence and Narrow Band Imaging in Barrett's Esophagus

Lorenza Alvarez Herrero, MD[a,b], Bas L.A.M. Weusten, MD, PhD[a,b], Jacques J.G.H.M. Bergman, MD, PhD[b],*

KEYWORDS

- Barrett's esophagus • Esophageal neoplasms
- Autofluorescence • Narrow band imaging
- Magnification endoscopy • Advanced imaging

Barrett's esophagus is a premalignant condition with an estimated annual cancer risk of 0.5%.[1] Esophageal adenocarcinoma is known to develop through a multistep transition sequence starting with nonneoplastic Barrett's epithelium, continuing through low-grade intraepithelial neoplasia (LGIN) and high-grade intraepithelial neoplasia (HGIN), and finally progressing into invasive early neoplasia (EN).[2] Patients with Barrett's esophagus are offered regular surveillance endoscopies to detect neoplasia at an early and curable stage. Present guidelines advise biopsy of the Barrett's epithelium according to the Seattle protocol, whereby biopsies are obtained from any visible abnormality in addition to 4-quadrant random biopsies taken every 2 cm.[3,4] This approach is, however, associated with sampling error because neoplastic lesions are often poorly visible and random biopsies only sample a small part of the Barrett's esophagus. Furthermore, biopsying in 4 quadrants every 2 cm is time consuming, leading to low protocol adherence by endoscopists in daily practice.[5,6]

In recent years, new imaging techniques have been developed to improve the detection of (intraepithelial) neoplasia at an early stage, thereby possibly improving Barrett's surveillance practice. These imaging techniques can mainly be divided into 2 types: detection techniques and characterization techniques. Detection imaging techniques are developed to serve as red flag techniques to improve the detection of (intraepithelial) neoplasia by drawing attention to lesions that may harbor early stages of (intraepithelial) neoplasia. A detection imaging technique is typically used

Disclosure: Jacques J.G.H.M. Bergman receives financial support from Olympus, Tokyo, Japan.
[a] Department of Gastroenterology and Hepatology, Sint Antonius Hospital, Koekoekslaan 1, 3430 EM, Nieuwegein, The Netherlands
[b] Department of Gastroenterology and Hepatology, Academic Medical Center, Meibergdreef 9, 1105 AZ, Amsterdam, The Netherlands
* Corresponding author.
E-mail address: j.j.bergman@amc.uva.nl

0889-8553/10/$ – see front matter © 2010 Elsevier Inc. All rights reserved.

during broad field overview examination in addition to white light endoscopy. Characterization imaging techniques, on the other hand, are meant for detailed inspection of detected lesions to characterize the lesion and to differentiate between neoplastic and nonneoplastic lesions. In general, characterization techniques are used on a small area by zooming in on the mucosa to provide more details.

This review discusses the application of 2 novel imaging techniques in Barrett's esophagus: autofluorescence and narrow band imaging (NBI).

AUTOFLUORESCENCE
Principle and Technique

Autofluorescence is the phenomenon in which tissue, after exposure to light of a certain wavelength, emits light of a longer wavelength. In tissue, endogenous fluorophores (eg, collagen, amino acids, flavins, nicotinamide adenine dinucleotide, and porphyrins) emit fluorescent light with a longer wavelength (ie, green and red light) after exposure to the short wavelength light (ie, ultraviolet or blue light). Besides initiating autofluorescence, short wavelength light can also be reflected, scattered, and absorbed by the tissues. Absorption of (fluorescent) light is possible by chromophores. The main chromophore in the gastrointestinal tissue that absorbs light in the visible wavelength (400–700 nm) is hemoglobin.

Compositional changes of the endogenous fluorophores and chromophores and stromal changes such as the thickening of the mucosa can influence the wavelength and intensity of the emitted autofluorescent light. Because of these changes, neoplastic lesions can exhibit an autofluorescent pattern that is different from that of normal tissue. Studies using point spectroscopy techniques, with small probes inserted through the accessory channel of the endoscope, have shown that the autofluorescence pattern of Barrett's neoplasia is different from that of normal Barrett's mucosa.[7–9] This difference in autofluorescence in Barrett's neoplasia is, however, believed to be mainly caused by changes in the stroma and hemoglobin concentration rather than changes in fluorophores composition.[10]

The Light Induced Fluorescence Endoscopy (LIFE) system (Xillix Technologies, Richmond, British Columbia, Canada) was the first endoscopy system that enabled autofluorescent imaging as a broad field technique. This system consisted of a camera mounted on the ocular portion of a fiberoptic endoscope. Switching between the white light mode and the autofluorescence mode was possible by using the switch on the camera. After excitation with blue light, the emitted red and green autofluorescent light passed from 2 charge coupled devices in the camera to the image processor. Based on the ratio of red to green autofluorescence, the image processor produced a real-time endoscopic image on a monitor using pseudocolors. Concurrently with LIFE, another comparable system from another manufacturer was also available (Storz, Tuttlingen, Germany).

The major problem with these systems was the use of fiberoptic endoscopy, which had a much lower resolution than the current video endoscopy systems. A new AFI system (Olympus, Tokyo, Japan) was therefore developed, consisting of a sequential red, green, and blue light source and a high-resolution video endoscope. Changing between the high-resolution white light mode and the AFI mode was made easy by pushing a control button on the endoscope. After excitation with blue light, a real-time AFI image was produced based on 3 light features: total emitted autofluorescence, green reflectance (540–560 nm), and red reflectance (600–620 nm). This was a more extended algorithm than LIFE, which only used the ratio of red to green autofluorescence.

Finally, the endoscopic trimodal imaging (ETMI) system (Olympus, Tokyo, Japan) was developed, which is currently commercially available in Asia and the United Kingdom.

ETMI is comparable with the AFI system but has additional features when using the high-resolution white light mode, during which NBI and optical zoom (magnification up to ×100) are possible. Most importantly, the algorithm of the autofluorescence mode was changed. The autofluorescence image is composed of 2 instead of 3 light features: total emitted autofluorescence and green reflectance (540–560 nm). Similar to the other systems, these light features are displayed as pseudocolors on the real-time endoscopic image on the monitor. In the case of ETMI, normal Barrett's mucosa appears green, and (an area suspicious for) neoplasia is displayed as purple (**Fig. 1**).

Clinical Application

Detection of neoplasia in Barrett's mucosa

The first studies with the autofluorescence systems using fiberoptic endoscopy (the LIFE system) reported a higher detection rate of HGIN/EN with autofluorescence.[11,12] Further evaluation with randomized crossover studies comparing white light video endoscopy with autofluorescence using the LIFE system showed, however, that autofluorescence did not increase the number of patients detected with HGIN/EN.[13,14] Possible explanations for the lack of increased detection were the poor image quality of the fiberoptic endoscopy and the algorithm that did not take distorting effects into account.

Both problems were overcome when autofluorescence was translated to video endoscopy (AFI and ETMI), which had high-resolution endoscopy and a new algorithm. Feasibility studies with AFI and ETMI showed that after inspection with high-resolution white light, inspection with autofluorescence resulted in additional detection of lesions and patients with HGIN/EN.[15–17] The targeted detection of patients with HGIN/EN increased from 43% to 65% after inspection with high-resolution white light and up to 90% to 100% after additional inspection with autofluorescence. The major drawback of autofluorescence was the high false-positive rate, as 40% to 81% of the lesions detected with autofluorescence did not contain HGIN/EN.[15–17]

A recent randomized crossover study comparing ETMI with standard video endoscopy showed that targeted detection was significantly better with ETMI: 65% versus 44% with standard video endoscopy.[18] Overall detection of the patients with HGIN/EN using ETMI (ie, targeted and random biopsies), however, was not statistically different from standard video endoscopy (84% vs 73%, respectively).[18] Furthermore, random

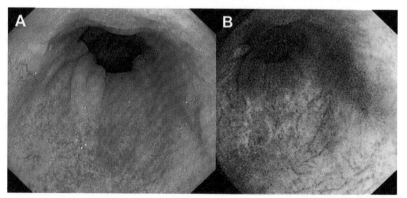

Fig. 1. Autofluorescence image of a Barrett's esophagus with corresponding high-resolution white light image. Neoplastic Barrett's mucosa (*A, B*) appears purple at the 3-o'clock position with autofluorescence (*B*).

biopsies resulted in the detection of additional patients with HGIN/EN (64% with targeted biopsies vs 84% with targeted and random biopsies), which suggests that improved targeted imaging with ETMI is not enough to abandon random biopsy sampling. Finally, a high number of lesions detected with ETMI were false-positive results (71%), although standard video endoscopy showed a high false-positive rate as well (53%). This study was performed by endoscopists with extensive expertise in imaging and endoscopic treatment of Barrett's esophagus, and only patients referred for HGIN/EN were included, that is, the study was performed in a high-risk population (with a high pretest likelihood of having HGIN/EN) by endoscopists who were used to see subtle lesions with HGIN/EN.

Hence, although autofluorescence did not lead to the identification of more patients with HGIN/EN in a tertiary referral setting, its use in a community hospital setting might be of additional value. Therefore, a randomized crossover study comparing ETMI with standard video endoscopy was performed in patients with an intermediate risk (ie, LGIN) by endoscopists without specific expertise in Barrett's esophagus.[19] Similar to the tertiary referral setting, the targeted detection of LGIN/HGIN/EN was again significantly increased with ETMI compared with standard video endoscopy (54% and 34%, respectively), but overall detection rates of patients with neoplastic changes in their Barrett's esophagus were not significantly different. False-positive rates remained high with ETMI (68%) as well as with standard video endoscopy (64%).[19]

Therefore, autofluorescence seems to increase the targeted detection of HGIN/EN lesions, although it does not result in a better overall detection of patients with HGIN/EN. The increased targeted detection rate might be useful to direct endoscopic therapy, although studies on this subject are lacking. Interobserver agreement on autofluorescence also seems to be reasonable with a kappa (κ) value of 0.48 to 0.76.[20,21] Still, the false-positive rate of autofluorescence remains a drawback.

Attempts to reduce the false-positive rate have been made by inspecting autofluorescent positive areas in detail with NBI. The false-positive rate was substantially reduced after NBI inspection from 40%–81% to 10%–48%.[16–19] This reduction in false-positive rates, however, was achieved at the expense of misclassifying a significant proportion (8%–17%) of the autofluorescent true positive areas as nonneoplastic.[16–19]

The endoscopic features associated with true positive autofluorescent areas (ie, autofluorescent positive areas containing HGIN/EN) were therefore studied to reduce the false-positive rate of autofluorescence. Opaque autofluorescent intensity, a different appearance of the area after reinspection with white light, and no close proximity to gastric folds (>1 cm) were found to be associated with true positive autofluorescent lesions. Although further evaluation is needed, these endoscopic features may be helpful in improving the accuracy of autofluorescence.[20]

In summary, autofluorescence increases the targeted detection of lesions with HGIN/EN and may therefore be useful in a tertiary center setting to direct endoscopic therapy. Autofluorescence, however, does not result in a better overall detection of patients with HGIN/EN. Furthermore, the false-positive rate of autofluorescence remains a major drawback.

NBI
Principle and Technique

NBI is a technique that uses optical filters to visualize the mucosal morphology by enhancing the mucosal as well as vascular patterns. NBI is based on the fact that the depth of light penetration into tissues depends on the wavelength of the light. Long wavelength light (red) penetrates deeper into tissue than short wavelength light (blue). Consequently, red light provides more information on the deeper layers of the mucosa, whereas blue light, which has a more superficial penetration, provides more information on the morphology of the mucosal surface. In addition, blue light reveals the superficial vasculature because it is absorbed by hemoglobin. With NBI, the relative intensity of the blue light is increased, whereas other wavelengths are reduced or eliminated by using a filter with narrow bandpass ranges.[22]

Other techniques that enhance the mucosal morphology during real-time endoscopy, such as Fuji Intelligent Color Enhancement (FICE) (Fujinon Inc, Saitama, Japan) and i-Scan (Pentax, Tokyo, Japan), are also available. These techniques differ from NBI in that they are postprocessing techniques. These techniques do not use actual filters but change the white light endoscopic image from the video processor by arithmetically processing it into a virtual image for different wavelength settings.[23,24] Studies using these techniques for Barrett's esophagus are rare (FICE) or lacking (I-scan).[25] Consequently, most data are known from studies that have been performed with NBI.

NBI is easy to use during endoscopy. Changing between the white light mode and the NBI mode on the endoscope is achieved by using a switch on the endoscope that deploys the NBI filter. NBI can be used during overview examination as a detection technique or for detailed inspection of mucosal and vascular patterns as a characterization modality.

Clinical Applications

Detection of neoplasia in Barrett's mucosa

The value of NBI for the detection of HGIN/EN is unclear. Two studies have reported on the use of NBI for the detection of (intraepithelial) neoplasia in Barrett's esophagus.[26,27] Kara and colleagues[26] evaluated the additional value of NBI and indigo carmine chromoendoscopy (ICC) and compared it with high-resolution white light endoscopy performed by endoscopists with specific expertise in Barrett's esophagus in patients referred with endoscopically inconspicuous HGIN/EN. A total of 28 patients underwent 2 endoscopies at an interval of 6 to 8 weeks, one with high-resolution white light endoscopy followed by NBI and the other with high-resolution white light endoscopy followed by ICC. NBI, as well as ICC, did not result in the additional detection of patients with HGIN/EN. Nevertheless, NBI, as well as ICC, resulted in the detection of a limited number of additional lesions with HGIN/EN in patients in whom high-resolution white light endoscopy already detected neoplasia. Wolfsen and colleagues[27] evaluated the detection rate of (intraepithelial) neoplasia with NBI and compared it with that of standard resolution white light in 65 patients referred for evaluation of (intraepithelial) neoplasia or enrolled in Barrett's surveillance. Patients underwent 1 endoscopy, first inspected with standard resolution white light endoscopy by one endoscopist, followed by high-resolution white light endoscopy and NBI performed by a second endoscopist. NBI detected significantly more patients with higher grades of (intraepithelial) neoplasia than standard resolution white light endoscopy. However, some limitations may have biased the results. First, the standard resolution white light endoscopy was performed by a group of endoscopists, whereas the NBI endoscopy was restricted to 2 endoscopists with experience in advanced endoscopy. The NBI endoscopy included inspection with high-resolution white light endoscopy, which may be at least as important as NBI alone for the detection of neoplasia. In addition, NBI endoscopy inspection time was twice as long as that of standard endoscopy because the Barrett's esophagus was inspected twice: once with high-resolution white light endoscopy and once with NBI.[28]

Clearly, further studies are needed to determine if NBI is useful during overview examination for the detection of (intraepithelial) neoplasia in Barrett's esophagus.

Characterization of Barrett's neoplasia

When using NBI with zoom, mucosal and vascular patterns can be inspected in detail. Mucosal morphology has been described and classified by several study groups to differentiate (intraepithelial) neoplasia from nonneoplastic tissue.[29–31] Generally, regular or normal patterns are considered to be associated with nonneoplastic Barrett's mucosa, whereas irregular or abnormal patterns are considered to be associated with neoplasia (**Fig. 2, Table 1**). Most of the studies have been performed by blinded image evaluation: endoscopists scoring the NBI zoom images were blinded for the endoscopic overview information.[29,30,32–34] Other studies have been performed real time by freezing an NBI zoom image of a suspected area found during (autofluorescence) endoscopy.[16–19] The sensitivity to differentiate HGIN/EN from LGIN/nonneoplastic tissue has been reported to be 71% to 100%, with a specificity of 33% to 99%.[16–19,29,30,32–38] The sensitivity to differentiate LGIN/HGIN/EN from nonneoplastic tissue has been reported to be 59% to 89%, with a specificity of 36% to 72%.[19,30,34,35] Although initial studies were promising, subsequent studies showed a rather moderate sensitivity. Possibly, NBI zoom provides too much detail without apparent clinically relevant information, which might confuse endoscopists more than providing them with valuable information.[33]

The ability to differentiate neoplastic from nonneoplastic lesions by NBI zoom was not influenced by the endoscopist's expertise, as no clear differences were found between endoscopists with extensive experience in Barrett's imaging and endoscopists without special interest in Barrett's.[32–35]

Another important aspect in this respect is the agreement between endoscopists on the mucosal morphology with NBI. Interobserver agreement (ie, agreement between different endoscopists) has been reported to be fair to moderate according to Landis and Koch[39] (κ 0.39–0.59).[32–34,36] Intraobserver agreement (ie, agreement between the same endoscopist) has been reported to be slightly higher with a κ value between 0.60 and 0.62, which is moderate to substantial.[34] Surprisingly, interobserver and intraobserver agreement did not differ between endoscopists without extensive experience in Barrett's esophagus and expert endoscopists from tertiary referral centers.[32–34] Characterization of Barrett's lesions with NBI is thus disappointing, with a relatively low sensitivity and moderate agreement between endoscopists with and without extensive experience in Barrett's esophagus. In addition, all studies used still images that were obtained by experienced endoscopists, and images of inferior quality were excluded by most studies. In daily practice,

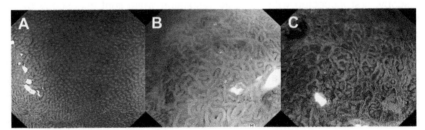

Fig. 2. (*A*) Narrow band imaging of mucosa in the cardia with round pits. (*B*) Barrett's mucosa with a more complicated branching pattern. (*C*) Irregular/abnormal appearing Barrett's mucosa containing neoplasia.

Table 1

Classifications on mucosal morphology to differentiate (intraepithelial) neoplasia from nonneoplastic tissue in Barrett's esophagus

Sharma et al[29]	Kara et al[30]	Herrero et al[34]	Anagnostopoulos et al[31]	Singh et al[35]
Mucosal pattern	Mucosal pattern	Mucosal pattern	Microstructural pattern	Microstructural or microvascular pattern
Circular	Regular	Regular	Round	Round pits & regular mv (pattern A)
Ridge/villous	Flat		Linear/tubular/villous	Villous/ridge pits & regular mv (pattern B)
–			Flat	Absent pits & regular mv (pattern C)
			Nonstructural	
Irregular/distorted	Irregular	Irregular	Irregular	Distorted pits & irregular mv (pattern D)
Vascular pattern	Vascular pattern	Vascular pattern	Microvascular pattern	
Normal	Regular	Regular	Regular	–
Abnormal	Irregular	Irregular	Irregular	–
	Abnormal blood vessels			
–	Absent	–		–
–	Present	–		–

Regular or normal patterns are considered to be associated with nonneoplastic mucosa; irregular or abnormal patterns are considered to be associated with neoplasia.

Abbreviation: mv, microvasculature.

less-experienced endoscopists may encounter difficulties when trying to take a high-quality still zoom image for evaluation with NBI. Biopsying areas that are suspected to have neoplasia, therefore, not only may result in a more accurate diagnosis but also is probably faster and more practical than obtaining a good-quality NBI image of the area of interest.

Characterization of intestinal metaplasia

Different mucosal patterns have been described and classified to differentiate intestinal metaplasia from gastric mucosa. Generally, round and circular patterns are believed to be associated with gastric mucosa, whereas more complicated branching patterns are believed to be associated with intestinal metaplasia (see **Fig. 2**).[29,31,40,41] The sensitivity for identifying intestinal metaplasia has been reported to be 56% to 100%, with specificities varying from 77% to 95%.[29,31,40–42] Despite assessments having been performed by expert endoscopists, accuracy is not optimal. Analogous to the characterization of neoplasia, characterization of intestinal metaplasia is best achieved by retrieving biopsies for histologic assessment instead of inspection with NBI.

Other clinical applications

A different application of NBI in Barrett's esophagus is its use for the detection of minute (1–5 mm) islands of columnar epithelium that might remain after ablation therapy, such as radiofrequency ablation.[43,44] Detection of such islands may be difficult with high-resolution white light endoscopy, whereas NBI may reveal the islands more easily (**Fig. 3**). Detecting such islands might help to adequately direct further ablative therapy.[43–46]

Finally, NBI may help to better delineate early neoplastic lesions before endoscopic resection.[47,48]

SUMMARY AND FUTURE PERSPECTIVE

Autofluorescence does increase the targeted detection of lesions containing HGIN/EN and may therefore be useful in tertiary centers to adequately locate neoplastic lesions for further endoscopic treatment. Compared with the current Seattle biopsy protocol, however, autofluorescence does not result in the detection of more patients with HGIN/EN, and autofluorescence in its current form will not replace random biopsies. Whether NBI detects more patients with HGIN/EN compared with the Seattle protocol needs further evaluation because, to date, only 2 studies with conflicting results have investigated NBI for this purpose. NBI seems, however, not to be useful in the characterization of Barrett's neoplasia given the relatively low sensitivity, even in expert hands. Biopsying areas that are suspected to harbor neoplasia is more practical and results in a more accurate diagnosis. Although autofluorescence and NBI may help to direct endoscopic therapy for HGIN/EN in Barrett's esophagus, their current value in daily practice seems to be limited.

Nevertheless, there is room to improve both techniques. In the case of AFI, new algorithms as well as combination with fluorescent markers may improve the detection rate of neoplasia and reduce the rate of false positivity. In the case of NBI, studies have focused too much on the characterization of lesions by evaluating still images. This is an artificial setting, different from real-time video assessment. In addition, histology of the biopsies was used as a gold standard, which may be suboptimal. Studies have shown that endoscopic resection (ie, a larger sample) leads to upgrading of the histologic diagnosis in 34% of the cases when HGIN/EN is evaluated.[49] Most important, however, is the possibility that too much focus may be

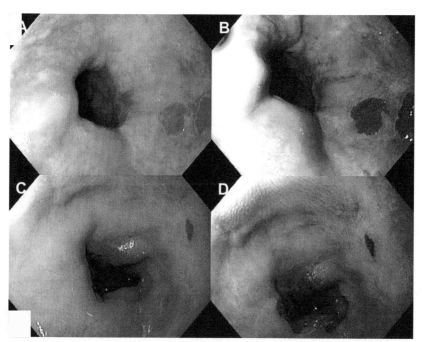

Fig. 3. Barrett's esophagus after radiofrequency ablation seen with high-resolution white light (*A, C*) and with narrow band imaging (*B, D*), in which the reaming islands of columnar epithelium are seen more clearly.

directed on high-magnification inspection by the evaluation of the mucosal and vascular patterns in detailed zoom. There may be other NBI features that are helpful in overview, such as surface relief, which might reveal neoplastic lesions more clearly in the Barrett's esophagus (**Fig. 4**).

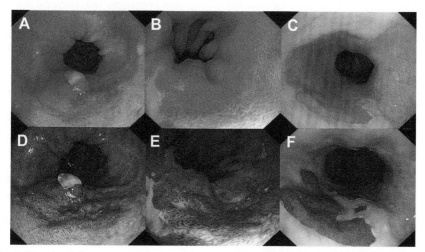

Fig. 4. Neoplastic lesions in Barrett's esophagus shown with high-resolution white light (*A–C*) and their corresponding images with narrow band imaging (*D–F*). Surface relief is better appreciated with narrow band imaging, which might aid in detecting more subtle lesions (*E, F*) or delineating them for endoscopic resection (*D*).

In summary, autofluorescence as well as NBI may be useful in directing endoscopic therapy for EN in Barrett's esophagus. Further research may reveal additional value for daily practice.

REFERENCES

1. Sharma P, Falk GW, Weston AP, et al. Dysplasia and cancer in a large multicenter cohort of patients with Barrett's esophagus. Clin Gastroenterol Hepatol 2006;4: 566–72.
2. Hameeteman W, Tytgat GN, Houthoff HJ, et al. Barrett's esophagus: development of dysplasia and adenocarcinoma. Gastroenterology 1989;96:1249–56.
3. Wang KK, Sampliner RE. Updated guidelines 2008 for the diagnosis, surveillance and therapy of Barrett's esophagus. Am J Gastroenterol 2008;103:788–97.
4. Hirota WK, Zuckerman MJ, Adler DG, et al. ASGE guideline: the role of endoscopy in the surveillance of premalignant conditions of the upper GI tract. Gastrointest Endosc 2006;63:570–80.
5. Curvers WL, Peters FP, Elzer B, et al. Quality of Barrett's surveillance in The Netherlands: a standardized review of endoscopy and pathology reports. Eur J Gastroenterol Hepatol 2008;20:601–7.
6. Abrams JA, Kapel RC, Lindberg GM, et al. Adherence to biopsy guidelines for Barrett's esophagus surveillance in the community setting in the United States. Clin Gastroenterol Hepatol 2009;7:736–42.
7. Panjehpour M, Overholt BF, Vo-Dinh T, et al. Endoscopic fluorescence detection of high-grade dysplasia in Barrett's esophagus. Gastroenterology 1996;111: 93–101.
8. Bourg-Heckly G, Blais J, Padilla JJ, et al. Endoscopic ultraviolet-induced autofluorescence spectroscopy of the esophagus: tissue characterization and potential for early cancer diagnosis. Endoscopy 2000;32:756–65.
9. Georgakoudi I, Jacobson BC, Van DJ, et al. Fluorescence, reflectance, and light-scattering spectroscopy for evaluating dysplasia in patients with Barrett's esophagus. Gastroenterology 2001;120:1620–9.
10. Kara MA, DaCosta RS, Streutker CJ, et al. Characterization of tissue autofluorescence in Barrett's esophagus by confocal fluorescence microscopy. Dis Esophagus 2007;20:141–50.
11. Haringsma J, Tytgat GN, Yano H, et al. Autofluorescence endoscopy: feasibility of detection of GI neoplasms unapparent to white light endoscopy with an evolving technology. Gastrointest Endosc 2001;53:642–50.
12. Niepsuj K, Niepsuj G, Cebula W, et al. Autofluorescence endoscopy for detection of high-grade dysplasia in short-segment Barrett's esophagus. Gastrointest Endosc 2003;58:715–9.
13. Kara MA, Smits ME, Rosmolen WD, et al. A randomized crossover study comparing light-induced fluorescence endoscopy with standard videoendoscopy for the detection of early neoplasia in Barrett's esophagus. Gastrointest Endosc 2005;61:671–8.
14. Borovicka J, Fischer J, Neuweiler J, et al. Autofluorescence endoscopy in surveillance of Barrett's esophagus: a multicenter randomized trial on diagnostic efficacy. Endoscopy 2006;38:867–72.
15. Kara MA, Peters FP, ten Kate FJ, et al. Endoscopic video autofluorescence imaging may improve the detection of early neoplasia in patients with Barrett's esophagus. Gastrointest Endosc 2005;61:679–85.

16. Kara MA, Peters FP, Fockens P, et al. Endoscopic video-autofluorescence imaging followed by narrow band imaging for detecting early neoplasia in Barrett's esophagus. Gastrointest Endosc 2006;64:176–85.
17. Curvers WL, Singh R, Wong Kee Song LM, et al. Endoscopic tri-modal imaging for detection of early neoplasia in Barrett's oesophagus; a multi-centre feasibility study using high-resolution endoscopy, autofluorescence imaging and narrow band imaging incorporated in one endoscopy system. Gut 2007;57:167–72.
18. Curvers WL, Herrero LA, Wallace MB, et al. Endoscopic Tri-Modal Imaging improves targeted detection of early neoplasia in Barrett's esophagus in a high-risk population; an international multi-center randomized cross-over study. Gastroenterology 2010 [online].
19. Curvers WL, van Vilsteren FG, Baak BC, et al. A multi-centre randomized cross-over trial comparing endoscopic tri-modal imaging (ETMI) with standard endoscopy (SE) for the detection of dysplasia in Barrett's esophagus (BE) patients with confirmed LGD performed in a non-university setting. Gastroenterology 2010;138:S155.
20. Curvers WL, Singh R, Wallace MB, et al. Identification of predictive factors for early neoplasia in Barrett's esophagus after autofluorescence imaging: a stepwise multicenter structured assessment. Gastrointest Endosc 2009;70:9–17.
21. Kim RE, Singh V, Hall SB, et al. Use of video-autofluorescence imaging (AFI) and magnification narrow band imaging (zoom-NBI) in Barrett's esophagus: an Inter-Observer Agreement Study. Gastrointest Endosc 2010;71:AB203.
22. Gono K, Obi T, Yamaguchi M, et al. Appearance of enhanced tissue features in narrow-band endoscopic imaging. J Biomed Opt 2004;9:568–77.
23. Pohl J, May A, Rabenstein T, et al. Computed virtual chromoendoscopy: a new tool for enhancing tissue surface structures. Endoscopy 2007;39:80–3.
24. Hoffman A, Basting N, Goetz M, et al. High-definition endoscopy with i-Scan and Lugol's solution for more precise detection of mucosal breaks in patients with reflux symptoms. Endoscopy 2009;41:107–12.
25. Pohl J, May A, Rabenstein T, et al. Comparison of computed virtual chromoendoscopy and conventional chromoendoscopy with acetic acid for detection of neoplasia in Barrett's esophagus. Endoscopy 2007;39:594–8.
26. Kara MA, Peters FP, Rosmolen WD, et al. High-resolution endoscopy plus chromoendoscopy or narrow-band imaging in Barrett's esophagus: a prospective randomized crossover study. Endoscopy 2005;37:929–36.
27. Wolfsen HC, Crook JE, Krishna M, et al. Prospective, controlled tandem endoscopy study of narrow band imaging for dysplasia detection in Barrett's esophagus. Gastroenterology 2008;135:24–31.
28. Curvers WL, Bergman JJ. Multimodality imaging in Barrett's esophagus: looking longer, seeing better, and recognizing more. Gastroenterology 2008;135:24–31.
29. Sharma P, Bansal A, Mathur S, et al. The utility of a novel narrow band imaging endoscopy system in patients with Barrett's esophagus. Gastrointest Endosc 2006;64:167–75.
30. Kara MA, Ennahachi M, Fockens P, et al. Detection and classification of the mucosal and vascular patterns (mucosal morphology) in Barrett's esophagus by using narrow band imaging. Gastrointest Endosc 2006;64:155–66.
31. Anagnostopoulos GK, Yao K, Kaye P, et al. Novel endoscopic observation in Barrett's oesophagus using high resolution magnification endoscopy and narrow band imaging. Aliment Pharmacol Ther 2007;26:501–7.
32. Curvers WL, Bohmer C, Mallant-Hent RC, et al. Mucosal morphology in Barrett's esophagus: inter-observer agreement and role of narrow band imaging. Endoscopy 2008;40:799–805.

33. Curvers W, Baak L, Kiesslich R, et al. Chromoendoscopy and narrow-band imaging compared with high-resolution magnification endoscopy in Barrett's esophagus. Gastroenterology 2008;134:670–9.

34. Herrero LA, Curvers WL, Bansal A, et al. Zooming in on Barrett oesophagus using narrow-band imaging: an international observer agreement study. Eur J Gastroenterol Hepatol 2009;21:1068–75.

35. Singh R, Anagnostopoulos GK, Yao K, et al. Narrow-band imaging with magnification in Barrett's esophagus: validation of a simplified grading system of mucosal morphology patterns against histology. Endoscopy 2008;40:457–63.

36. Singh R, Karageorgiou H, Owen V, et al. Comparison of high-resolution magnification narrow-band imaging and white-light endoscopy in the prediction of histology in Barrett's oesophagus. Scand J Gastroenterol 2009;44:85–92.

37. Curvers WL, van den Broek FJ, Reitsma JB, et al. Systematic review of narrow-band imaging for the detection and differentiation of abnormalities in the esophagus and stomach (with video). Gastrointest Endosc 2009;69:307–17.

38. Mannath J, Subramanian V, Hawkey CJ, et al. Narrow band imaging for characterization of high grade dysplasia and specialized intestinal metaplasia in Barrett's esophagus: a meta-analysis. Endoscopy 2010;42:351–9.

39. Landis JR, Koch GG. The measurement of observer agreement for categorical data. Biometrics 1977;33:159–74.

40. Hamamoto Y, Endo T, Nosho K, et al. Usefulness of narrow-band imaging endoscopy for diagnosis of Barrett's esophagus. J Gastroenterol 2004;39:14–20.

41. Goda K, Tajiri H, Ikegami M, et al. Usefulness of magnifying endoscopy with narrow band imaging for the detection of specialized intestinal metaplasia in columnar-lined esophagus and Barrett's adenocarcinoma. Gastrointest Endosc 2007;65:36–46.

42. Norimura D, Isomoto H, Nakayama T, et al. Magnifying endoscopic observation with narrow band imaging for specialized intestinal metaplasia in Barrett's esophagus with special reference to light blue crests. Dig Endosc 2010;22:101–6.

43. Gondrie JJ, Pouw RE, Sondermeijer CM, et al. Stepwise circumferential and focal ablation of Barrett's esophagus with high-grade dysplasia: results of the first prospective series of 11 patients. Endoscopy 2008;40:359–69.

44. Gondrie JJ, Pouw RE, Sondermeijer CM, et al. Effective treatment of early Barrett's neoplasia with stepwise circumferential and focal ablation using the HALO system. Endoscopy 2008;40:370–9.

45. Pouw RE, Gondrie JJ, Sondermeijer CM, et al. Eradication of Barrett esophagus with early neoplasia by radiofrequency ablation, with or without endoscopic resection. J Gastrointest Surg 2008;12:1627–36.

46. Pouw RE, Wirths K, Eisendrath P, et al. Efficacy of radiofrequency ablation combined with endoscopic resection for Barrett's esophagus with early neoplasia. Clin Gastroenterol Hepatol 2009;8:23–9.

47. Kadowaki S, Tanaka K, Toyoda H, et al. Ease of early gastric cancer demarcation recognition: a comparison of four magnifying endoscopy methods. J Gastroenterol Hepatol 2009;24:1625–30.

48. Thomas T, Singh R, Ragunath K. Trimodal imaging-assisted endoscopic mucosal resection of early Barrett's neoplasia. Surg Endosc 2009;23:1609–13.

49. Hull MJ, Mino-Kenudson M, Nishioka NS, et al. Endoscopic mucosal resection: an improved diagnostic procedure for early gastroesophageal epithelial neoplasms. Am J Surg Pathol 2006;30:114–8.

Endomicroscopy of Barrett's Esophagus

Marcia Irene Canto, MD, MHS

KEYWORDS

• Barrett's esophagus • Confocal laser endomicroscopy
• eCLE • pCLE

Histopathologic examination of formalin-fixed hematoxylin-eosin stained mucosal specimens has been the reference diagnostic standard for gastroenterology. In the last decade, it has become possible to perform virtual histology during gastrointestinal endoscopy through the miniaturization of a laser scanning microscope with confocal optics. High-resolution microscopic images are generated by illuminating the area of interest with a low power argon blue laser (488 nm) and collecting the reflected fluorescence through a small aperture. Confocal pinhole imaging enables rejection of out-of-focus laser light and computer-based reconstruction to generate an optical section of the tissue at a specific depth or plane. The microscopic images of the mucosa are collected at a fixed depth (probe-based confocal laser endomicroscopy [pCLE]) or at multiple but limited depths from the surface (endoscope-based confocal laser endomicroscopy [eCLE]).

Confocal laser endomicroscopy is a technique that involves a scanning laser light coupled with a fluorescent agent to generate highly magnified microscopic images of the gastrointestinal mucosa. CLE without use of a contrast agent was first reported by Japanese investigators in 2003[1] when a CLE probe prototype was used ex vivo in resected colon specimens and in vivo in one healthy volunteer to visualize colonic mucosa. The first use of contrast-aided CLE was reported by Kiesslich and colleagues[2] from Mainz, Germany. Using both acriflavine and fluorescein, the investigators reported a highly accurate prediction of colonic neoplasia.

ENDOMICROSCOPY PLATFORMS AND EQUIPMENT

There are currently 2 confocal endomicroscopy systems available: a confocal endoscope (eCLE), the EC3870CILK (Pentax, Tokyo, Japan), and a probe-based confocal endomicroscopy (pCLE), the Cellvizio (Mauna Kea Technologies, Paris, France).

Division of Gastroenterology and Hepatology, Department of Medicine, Johns Hopkins University School of Medicine, 1830 East Monument Street, Room 427, Baltimore, MD 21205, USA
E-mail address: mcanto@jhmi.edu

Gastroenterol Clin N Am 39 (2010) 759–769
doi:10.1016/j.gtc.2010.08.032
0889-8553/10/$ – see front matter © 2010 Elsevier Inc. All rights reserved.

Both the eCLE and pCLE systems allow visualization of microscopic cellular and vascular patterns. **Table 1** details the technical aspects of each system and highlights the differences. For eCLE, a gastroscope EG-3870CILK and colonoscope 3870CIFK are available (Pentax, Tokyo, Japan). These endomicroscopes connect to a standard Pentax processor (for endoscopy) as well as the endomicroscopy computer processor. The current endoscopes are outfitted with standard-resolution white light optics. The shorter gastroscope-endomicroscope has centimeter markings at the distal end to facilitate measurements of distance of the endoscope tip from patients' teeth. The buttons, wheels, accessory channel, air-water and suction valves, shaft diameter (12.8 mm), and handling of the endomicroscope are similar to a videocolono- scope. The endomicroscope provides submicron resolution with a large field of view (see **Table 1**) of 475 µm × 475 µm. Furthermore, the direction of scanning and depth of imaging are controlled by buttons at the endoscope head and allow subsurface detailed analyses or continued imaging within the same plane/depth from the surface. The eCLE can be combined with chromoendoscopy for additional mucosal enhance- ment. Finally, the scanning speed can be varied from slow or 0.8 images per second (with higher resolution 1024 × 1024 pixel images generated) or fast rate (1.6 images per second [with 1024 × 512 pixel images]).

For the pCLE system, the Cellvizio system can be used with a variety of miniprobes that can be passed through the endoscope accessory channel (**Fig. 1**). These minip- robes come in different lengths for use in the upper gastrointestinal (GI) tract, colon, and bile duct. The lateral resolution of the different probes also varies (see **Table 1**) such that the probes with the highest resolution (1 µm) have a smaller field of view (240 µm) and the lower resolution probes (3.5 µm) have larger fields of view. The imaging depth is fixed for a particular probe. Importantly, the probe-based micro- scopic system enables flexibility of use with any endoscope and coupling of high- resolution endoscopy with other digital mucosal enhancements, such as narrow band imaging (Olympus Tokyo, Japan), IScan (Pentax, Tokyo, Japan), or FICE (Fujinon Tokyo, Japan). Scanning speed for the confocal microscope probes is 12 images per second, similar to video. Software enhancements allow stitching of the confocal images into a mosaic, which allows inspection of a wider field of the mucosa within the same plan. Confocal probes have a limited number of uses, which increases cost.

Both CLE systems allow image capture, storage, magnification, and export using either Windows-based (eCLE) or Macintosh-based (pCLE) computer systems. Management of CLE images is important for intraprocedure and postprocedure review. Both systems currently do not have a scroll function or cine-loop of images,

Table 1 Features of the available endomicroscopy systems				
	Endoscope (eCLE)	Probe (pCLE)		
Company	Pentax	Mauna Kea Technologies		
Devices	Upper endoscope colonoscope	Gastro/ Coloflex	Gastro/ Coloflex UHD	Cholangioflex
Imaging depth (µm)	0–250	70–130	55–65	40–70
Field of view (µm)	475 × 475	600	240	320
Lateral resolution (µm)	0.7	3.5	1.0	3.5
Axial resolution (µm)	7	15	5	—
Diameter (mm)	12.8	2.7	2.5	1.0

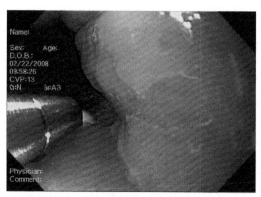

Fig. 1. Endoscopic image of confocal microscopic probe (Cellvizio, Mauna Kea Technologies) placed on Barrett's mucosa.

similar to that in endoscopic ultrasound systems. Magnification within captured images can facilitate visualization of minute subcellular and extracellular structures, such as Helicobacter pylori[3,4] and intramucosal bacteria.

CONTRAST AGENTS

Exogenous fluorescent contrast agents are currently necessary for endomicroscopic imaging using the commercially available single-photon systems. The natural fluorescence of the GI mucosa is not intense enough to allow detailed microscopic imaging, unlike autofluorescence imaging.

There are 2 general types of contrast agents: intravenous and topical. The most commonly used endomicroscopy contrast agent is intravenous fluorescein sodium. Fluorescein has been used for decades by ophthalmologists for imaging of the retinal vasculature. To date, it has not been approved by the US Food and Drug Administration (FDA) for use with CLE. Intravenous fluorescein sodium has been used for decades and has a high safety profile. Adverse events are rare. Other than yellowing of the skin, eyes, and urine in all patients that lasts several hours, complications with fluorescein are unusual. Based on a large multicenter retrospective study, the incidence of fluorescein-related adverse effects is 1.4%, including nausea, hypotension, rash, and injection site erythema.[5] Intravenous fluorescein highlights the vessels, intracellular spaces, and lamina propria, but does not stain nuclei. With fluorescein, intraepithelial mucin appears dark caused by acid pH. Hence, the hallmark of goblet cells in Barrett's esophagus (BE) (as well as those in the small bowel and colon) appears dark. Vessels and capillaries appear bright, and red blood cells can be seen as dark ovals. After injection of 2.5 to 5.0 mL of fluorescein, the epithelial cells should be readily visible. Fluorescein typically lasts about 30 minutes. Some endoscopists may start with 2.5 mL injection and give a second dose of 2.5 mL if needed for longer procedures.

Topical contrast agents, such as acriflavine and cresyl violet, can also be used during eCLE and pCLE. These two agents are also not specifically approved by the FDA for CLE. Acriflavine dye is a topical antiseptic and agent for freshwater and marine aquariums. In CLE, 0.05% acriflavine has been used as a contrast agent during endomicroscopy. Unlike fluorescein, it stains the nuclei of cells. It can be used in combination with fluorescein for maximum visualization of cellular and subcellular structures. Topical acriflavine has been used in the gastrointestinal tract to image H pylori, colon polyps,[2,4] oral and oropharyngeal mucosa,[6] and acute graft-versus-host disease in the colon . Outside the GI tract, it has been used in combination with acetic acid during cervical colposcopy to detect cervical intraepithelial neoplasia.[7] Acriflavine is used much less frequently because of concern about its mutagenic potential. Topical cresyl violet 0.25% to 1% is a dye that can also be used for chromoendoscopy.[8] Cresyl violet highlights the cytoplasm and enables visualization of nuclei.

ENDOMICROSCOPIC FEATURES OF BARRETT'S ESOPHAGUS AND ASSOCIATED NEOPLASIA

Kiesslich and others[9] from the University of Mainz first reported the application of eCLE in Barrett's esophagus and described the endomicroscopic features of normal squamous esophageal mucosa, gastric metaplasia, Barrett's esophagus (intestinal metaplasia), and Barrett's with neoplasia (high-grade dysplasia and cancer). Using histopathology as the gold standard, the classification system predicted the final diagnosis of BE with a sensitivity of 98.0%, specificity of 94.0%, and accuracy of 97.5%. Blinded, independent correlation of the CLE mucosal cellular and vascular patterns in the surface and deeper in the mucosa with histopathology led to the creation of a simple Confocal Barrett Classification system for predicting in vivo histology, which is widely used today (**Table 2**).

Nondysplastic BE has glands with variable-sized lumen and epithelial cells with a picket-fence appearance (aligned, with delineation of cell borders) and variable number of small oval-shaped dark cells (goblet cells) (**Figs. 2** and **3**). The key features of high-grade neoplasia/dysplasia and early adenocarcinoma are changes in the appearance of the intestinal metaplastic cells (cells appear dark and lose the regular columnar picket-fence appearance, which indirectly corresponds to a high nuclear-cytoplasmic ratio and pseudostratification or less of basal orientation of nuclei) and cellular architecture (irregularly shaped glands) (**Fig. 4**). In malignant BE, there may also be increased number, diameter, density of capillaries,[10] and fluorescein leakage (bright signal outside epithelial cells in the lamina propria) (see **Fig. 4**).

ENDOSCOPE-BASED ENDOMICROSCOPY AND BARRETT'S ESOPHAGUS

In a single-center, blinded, prospective study, Kiesslich and colleagues reported high accuracy, sensitivity, and specificity of eCLE when performed by experts (**Table 3**). The majority of neoplastic BE were associated with mucosal lesions (Ralf Kiesslich, personal communication 2006). The interobserver and intraobserver variability for prediction of histologic diagnoses was low with kappa scores of 0.843 and 0.892 (excellent agreement).

Another prospective single-center study by Trovato and colleagues[11] from Italy reported preliminary data from 39 subjects with gastroesophageal reflux disease and known BE undergoing surveillance. The investigators also reported high sensitivity of eCLE for prediction of BE and associated neoplasia (see **Table 3**). The interobserver agreement was also good (k = 0.74).

In 2009, Dunbar and colleagues[12] from The Johns Hopkins Hospital reported results of their single-center, blinded, randomized crossover trial for eCLE in Barrett's esophagus. They examined the diagnostic yield for BE neoplasia and actual mucosal biopsy reduction in subjects undergoing surveillance and in subjects with suspected endoscopically inapparent neoplasia.[12] Subjects with known esophageal cancer or confirmed localized neoplastic mucosal lesions were excluded. In this study, 23 subjects undergoing surveillance and 16 subjects with nonlocalized neoplasia underwent eCLE and standard endoscopy in a randomized order. All subjects enrolled had both eCLE and standard endoscopy with random biopsy. During standard endoscopy,

Table 2
Confocal Barrett classification system

Confocal Diagnosis	Vessel Architecture	Image Examples: Upper and Deeper Parts of the Mucosal Layer
Gastric type epithelium	Capillaries of regular shape only visible in deeper parts of the mucosal layer	
Barrett's epithelium	Subepithelial capillaries of regular shape beneath columnar lined epithelium visible in upper and deeper parts of the mucosal layer	
Neoplasia	Irregular capillaries visible in upper and deeper parts of the mucosal layer. Leakage of vessels leads to a heterogeneous and brighter signal intensity within the lamina propria	
	Cell Architecture	**Image Examples**
Gastric type epithelium	Regular columnar lined epithelium with round glandular openings and typical cobble stone appearance	
Barrett's epithelium	Columnar lined epithelium with in between dark mucin in goblet cells in upper parts of the mucosal layer. In deeper parts, villous like, dark shaped regular cylindrical Barrett's epithelial cells are present	
Neoplasia	Black cells with irregular apical and distal borders and shapes with high dark contrast to surrounded tissue	

Reprinted from Kiesslich R, Gossner L, Goetz M, et al. In vivo histology of Barrett's esophagus and associated neoplasia by confocal laser endomicroscopy. Clin Gastroenterol Hepatol 2006 Aug;4(8):979–87. Epub 2006 Jul 13; with permission from Elsevier.

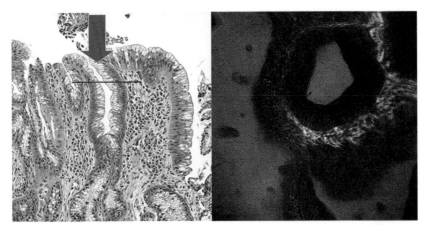

Fig. 2. Columnar epithelium with goblet cells (Barrett's esophagus). Right image obtained by confocal laser endomicroscopy acquired with the endomicroscope (Pentax) showing cross-sectional imaging of gland in the superficial mucosa. Left image shows histology of glandular epithelium of Barrett's esophagus with arrow indicating direction of CLE imaging perpendicular to the surface.

mucosal biopsies were obtained per standard of care according to the Seattle biopsy protocol. During eCLE, optical biopsies were acquired, but only targeted mucosal biopsies were obtained if the CLE imaging suggested neoplasia. Compared with standard endoscopy, eCLE with targeted mucosal biopsies increased the yield in subjects with unlocalized neoplasia from 17% to 34%. Furthermore, eCLE led to 59% fewer biopsies to achieve a comparable overall diagnosis (per subject analysis). Likewise, in subjects undergoing routine endoscopic surveillance, there were significantly less biopsies taken during CLE. Indeed, 65% of the subjects undergoing surveillance had no mucosal biopsies taken during CLE because their CLE imaging was normal.

Other investigators have also reported successful use of eCLE as "optical EMR (endoscopic mucosal resection)," enabling targeted EMR in subjects with long BE

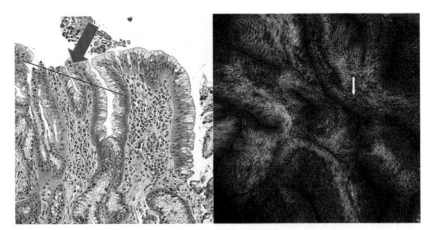

Fig. 3. Glandular epithelium of nondysplastic Barrett's esophagus with small oval-shaped dark goblet cells in uniformly aligned epithelial cells indicated with small down arrow (right image, endoscope-based endomicroscopy). Left image shows histology of glandular epithelium of Barrett's esophagus with arrow indicating direction of tangential CLE imaging.

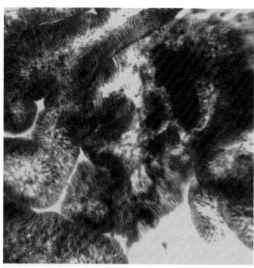

Fig. 4. Endomicroscopy image (obtained with Pentax endomicroscope after intravenous fluorescein) showing features of high-grade intraepithelial neoplasia and early invasive adenocarcinoma: dark epithelial cells, glandular distortion, increased number (density) of microvessels, and fluorescein extravasation at the center and right half of the image.

and unlocalized neoplasia.[13] In vivo eCLE imaging allowed localization of the focal high-grade dysplasia in flat BE mucosa and EMR immediately afterwards.

PROBE-BASED ENDOMICROSCOPY AND BARRETT'S ESOPHAGUS

Pohl and colleagues[14] from Germany reported the first pCLE study of Barrett's esophagus. In this 2-phase study, pCLE images were obtained from 15 subjects with BE and BE neoplasia and criteria for pCLE image characteristics were described. The pCLE criteria for BE and BE neoplasia were then used to evaluate pCLE images from 23 subjects to distinguish between dysplastic and nondysplastic BE. Two blinded investigators reviewed the images of BE and BE neoplasia. The in vivo sensitivity for detection of BE neoplasia was 75% with a specificity of 89% to 91%. The positive predictive value for BE neoplasia was 44% and the negative predictive value was 98% using pCLE, with good interobserver agreement (k = 0.6).

In a blinded multicenter study of 11 experts rating offline digital pCLE videos, Wallace and colleagues reported preliminary results for fluorescein-aided accuracy for BE after a training set of 20 images and test set of 20 images (11 with high-grade neoplasia or invasive cancer) (**Table 4**).

Table 3 Performance characteristics of eCLE for Barrett's esophagus and associated neoplasia		
	Prediction of Barrett's Esophagus	**Prediction of BE-Associated Neoplasia**
Kiesslich et al[9] 2006	Accuracy = 96.8% Sensitivity = 98.1% Specificity = 94.1%	Accuracy = 97.4% Sensitivity = 94.1% Specificity = 98.5%
Trovato et al[11] 2008	Sensitivity = 96.4%	

Table 4 Performance characteristics of pCLE for Barrett's esophagus and associated neoplasia	
Pohl et al[14] 2008	Sensitivity = 75%; specificity = 88.9% (rater 1) Sensitivity = 75%; specificity = 91.0% (rater 2)
Wallace et al[15] 2009	Sensitivity = 88%; specificity 96% (overall) Sensitivity = 91%; specificity 100% (with prior pCLE experience)
Bajbouj et al[16] 2010	Sensitivity = 12% (on site); 28% (blinded off site) Specificity = 95% (on site); 97% (blinded off site) Positive predictive value = 18% (on site); 46% (blinded off site) Negative predictive value = 92% (on site); 97% (blinded off site)

Recently in Germany, a 3-center blinded study reported a pCLE-guided, targeted mucosal biopsy versus 4-quadrant random biopsy in 63 subjects with both in vivo and offline interpretation of CLE (see **Table 3**).[16] Investigators used argon plasma coagulation to mark optical biopsy sites for the per biopsy analysis of accuracy. The overall prevalence of high-grade neoplasia or cancer was 8.3%, which was thought to be more representative of general gastroenterology practice. The sensitivity and positive predictive values for both in vivo and blinded interpretation of images were poor and the investigators concluded that pCLE-targeted biopsy may not yet replace standard biopsy techniques for surveillance of BE.

The potential factors associated with the pCLE accuracy rates of BE and associated neoplasia compared with eCLE could be lower resolution (particularly in early studies), smaller field of view, and motion artifact in probe-based images. The additive or complementary effects of enhanced mucosal imaging techniques, such as narrow band imaging, have not been reported.

TECHNIQUE FOR CLE IMAGING IN THE ESOPHAGUS AND GASTROESOPHAGEAL JUNCTION

Endomicroscopy should always be preceded by a careful examination of the mucosa with white light. Pay particular attention to the standard landmarks, the presence of any lesions, and presence of esophagitis. Wash away any thick mucus, food, or bubbles. Image lesions first, then perform the equivalent of a 4-quadrant biopsy from the different levels of BE. Although imaging of small islands and short tongues may be challenging, these areas need to be inspected because they may harbor high-grade neoplasia.

In general, the basic technique of endomicroscopy is not difficult, but imaging the esophagus and gastroesophageal junction is thought to be the most challenging because of esophageal motility, diaphragmatic movements, and oblique orientation of the esophageal mucosa. Stabilization of position is crucial. With eCLE, this is facilitated by application of gentle suction from the endoscope and anchoring the up-down wheel with the third digit of the left hand.

To obtain eCLE images, place the tip of the confocal endoscope directly on the mucosa, aiming for an en face position. The microscope window is located on the lower left portion of the endoscope tip and can be seen as a dark area at the left lower corner of the endoscopic image. The best images are obtained when the confocal imaging window is completely in contact against the mucosa. Apply suction to stabilize. Once a stable position is obtained, take time to inspect all areas of the CLE image within one plane before moving to deeper areas. Typically, columnar mucosa (including BE and gastric metaplasia in the esophagus) has greater vascularity (therefore epithelial cells appear brighter and are more readily visualized) than normal squamous epithelium. Hence, a few clicks moving downward from the surface into the superficial mucosa should lead to good visualization of BE. To calibrate and return the plane of imaging to the surface, press the home button (button 3). To begin sectioning down through the mucosa, press button 4. Holding button 4 down or pressing repeatedly will move the imaging plane 4 μm deeper into the mucosa. To reverse the direction of imaging, quickly press button 4 twice. Capture CLE images using the foot pedal (ideal), the mouse, or the touch screen. For beginners, scanning in the slower mode (1.6 images per second) may allow longer time for inspection and analysis of microscopic images. To biopsy an area imaged by eCLE, sample the area within 5 mm to the left of the suction polyp created during imaging, which will correspond to the position of the endomicroscope window.

The pCLE is technically easier to perform than eCLE. To perform pCLE, advance the probe through the endoscope channel and place the tip of the probe gently and directly on the surface of the mucosa with endoscopic guidance. The use of a plastic EMR cap attached to the end of the endoscope may help stabilize the pCLE image and decrease motion artifact. For flat neoplasia without associated mucosal abnormality, argon plasma coagulation may be needed to mark the area for EMR.

To learn endomicroscopy, it is ideal to perform at least some cases supervised by an endoscopist with training in endomicroscopy. Interpretation of endomicroscopic images from the esophagus may be initially challenging. Review of basic histology and routine review of endomicroscopic images in atlases and Web sites as well as routine comparison of CLE images with pathology images may help the endoscopist understand the differences in orientation of CLE and pathology images. Histology sections are made parallel to the mucosal surface and in vivo endomicroscopy optical sections are seen in perpendicular (or in cross section) or tangential/oblique orientation with regard to the mucosal surface (see **Figs. 2** and **3**).

POTENTIAL ROLE OF CLE IN GASTROENTEROLOGY PRACTICE

Endomicroscopy has the potential to impact clinical care and change the practice of gastroenterology. During endoscopy, it may localize neoplasia in the flat mucosa of BE or exclude the presence of it, which, in turn, may potentially decrease the number of biopsies of normal mucosa or obviate the need for mucosal sampling.[12] Targeted EMR is also an important clinical application for BE.[12,13] However, the exact role of endomicroscopy in relation to other available techniques of mucosal imaging, such as narrow band imaging and IScan, needs to be clarified. An ongoing multicenter, international, double-blind, randomized controlled trial may provide data on the accuracy, diagnostic yield, and clinical impact of eCLE after high-resolution white light endoscopy for imaging of suspected unlocalized BE neoplasia and routine surveillance of BE (www.clinicaltrials.gov).

FUTURE DIRECTIONS AND APPROACHES FOR ENDOMICROSCOPY

Commercially available CLE devices need improvement, including incorporation of high-resolution endoscopic imaging into the endomicroscope or further miniaturization of the microscope components with comparable lateral resolution to allow through-the-scope use.

CLE is not routinely available in most parts of the world. Apart from training, the high cost of equipment, the lack of a specific *Current Procedural Technology* code for billing, and FDA approval for fluorescein and other contrast agents in the United States are potential contributors to the slow adoption of this technology. Research on low-cost endoscopic microscopy suggests that there may be other alternatives to current

CLE devices available in the future. For example, a feasibility study of a low-cost fiber-optic endoscopic microscope reported detection of normal squamous, BE, and BE with high-grade dysplasia.[17] Development of dual photon fiberoptic laser microscopy[18] and spectrally encoded confocal microscopy[19] might one day eliminate the need for exogenous fluorescent contrast agents.

Molecular imaging using fluorescent-tagged molecules that attach to epithelial structures is also of great interest because it might eliminate the need for morphologic anatomic analysis and provide high specificity combined with a sensitive red-flag technique for broad scanning of large areas of mucosa, such as autofluorescence. Research on fluorescent peptide markers for BE using a similar approach as that reported for colonic adenomas[20] is ongoing in the United States.

SUMMARY

Endomicroscopy is a significant technological advance in gastrointestinal imaging that has been applied for in vivo diagnosis of BE and associated neoplasia. The eCLE has been shown to be highly accurate and potentially comparable to random biopsy for neoplasia detection. CLE has the potential to impact patient care. It needs to be studied in the context of practical and economic considerations. It should be used with high-resolution endoscopic techniques. To be routinely used in the care of patients with Barrett's esophagus and other GI diseases, it needs to be further developed to shift to noncontrast, high-resolution, low-cost probe-based imaging coupled with push-button digital red-flag mucosal enhancements.

REFERENCES

1. Sakashita M, Inoue H, Kashida H, et al. Virtual histology of colorectal lesions using laser-scanning confocal microscopy. Endoscopy 2003;35:1033–8.
2. Kiesslich R, Burg J, Vieth M, et al. Confocal laser endoscopy for diagnosing intraepithelial neoplasias and colorectal cancer in vivo. Gastroenterology 2004;127:706–13.
3. Ji R, Li YQ, Gu XM, et al. Confocal laser endomicroscopy for diagnosis of helicobacter pylori infection: a prospective study. J Gastroenterol Hepatol 2010;25:700–5.
4. Kiesslich R, Goetz M, Burg J, et al. Diagnosing helicobacter pylori in vivo by confocal laser endoscopy. Gastroenterology 2005;128:2119–23.
5. Wallace MB, Meining A, Canto MI, et al. The safety of intravenous fluorescein for confocal laser endomicroscopy in the gastrointestinal tract. Aliment Pharmacol Ther 2010;31:548–52.
6. Haxel BR, Goetz M, Kiesslich R, et al. Confocal endomicroscopy: a novel application for imaging of oral and oropharyngeal mucosa in human. Eur Arch Otorhinolaryngol 2010;267:443–8.
7. Tan J, Quinn MA, Pyman JM, et al. Detection of cervical intraepithelial neoplasia in vivo using confocal endomicroscopy. BJOG 2009;116:1663–70.
8. Goetz M, Toermer T, Vieth M, et al. Simultaneous confocal laser endomicroscopy and chromoendoscopy with topical cresyl violet. Gastrointest Endosc 2009;70:959–68.
9. Kiesslich R, Gossner L, Goetz M, et al. In vivo histology of Barrett's esophagus and associated neoplasia by confocal laser endomicroscopy. Clin Gastroenterol Hepatol 2006;4:979–87.

10. Becker V, Vieth M, Bajbouj M, et al. Confocal laser scanning fluorescence microscopy for in vivo determination of microvessel density in Barrett's esophagus. Endoscopy 2008;40:888–91.
11. Trovato C, Sonzogni A, Fiori G, et al. Confocal laser endomicroscopy for in-vivo diagnosis of Barrett's esophagus and associated neoplasia: an ongoing prospective study. Gastrointest Endosc 2008;67:AB97.
12. Dunbar KB, Okolo P 3rd, Montgomery E, et al. Confocal laser endomicroscopy in Barrett's esophagus and endoscopically inapparent Barrett's neoplasia: a prospective, randomized, double-blind, controlled, crossover trial. Gastrointest Endosc 2009;70:645–54.
13. Leung KK, Maru D, Abraham S, et al. Optical EMR: confocal endomicroscopy-targeted EMR of focal high-grade dysplasia in Barrett's esophagus. Gastrointest Endosc 2009;69:170–2.
14. Pohl H, Rosch T, Vieth M, et al. Miniprobe confocal laser microscopy for the detection of invisible neoplasia in patients with Barrett's oesophagus. Gut 2008; 57:1648–53.
15. Wallace MB, Sharma P, Lightdale C, et al. Preliminary accuracy and interobserver agreement for the detection of intraepithelial neoplasia in Barrett's esophagus with probe-based confocal laser endomicroscopy. Gastrointest Endosc 2010; 72:19–24.
16. Bajbouj M, Vieth M, Rosch T, et al. Probe-based confocal laser endomicroscopy compared with standard four-quadrant biopsy for evaluation of neoplasia in Barrett's esophagus. Endoscopy 2010;42:435–40.
17. Muldoon TJ, Anandasabapathy S, Maru D, et al. High-resolution imaging in Barrett's esophagus: a novel, low-cost endoscopic microscope. Gastrointest Endosc 2008;68:737–44.
18. Bao H, Boussioutas A, Reynolds J, et al. Imaging of goblet cells as a marker for intestinal metaplasia of the stomach by one-photon and two-photon fluorescence endomicroscopy. J Biomed Opt 2009;14:064031.
19. Kang D, Suter MJ, Boudoux C, et al. Comprehensive imaging of gastroesophageal biopsy samples by spectrally encoded confocal microscopy. Gastrointest Endosc 2010;71:35–43.
20. Hsiung PL, Hardy J, Friedland S, et al. Detection of colonic dysplasia in vivo using a targeted heptapeptide and confocal microendoscopy. Nat Med 2008;14:454–8.

High-Definition Endoscopy and Magnifying Endoscopy Combined with Narrow Band Imaging in Gastric Cancer

Mitsuru Kaise, MD, PhD[a],*, Masayuki Kato, MD, PhD[b],
Hisao Tajiri, MD, PhD[c]

KEYWORDS

- Gastric cancer • High-definition endoscopy
- Narrow band imaging • Magnifying endoscopy
- Autofluorescence endoscopy

Gastric cancer is the third common cancer and is the second leading cause of cancer deaths worldwide.[1] Because the high mortality from gastric cancer mainly results from late presentation in advanced stage of cancer with metastasis, efficacious screening and curative treatment at an early stage is one of the main ways to reduce gastric cancer death. Endoscopy is being increasingly used for gastric cancer screening because of a high detection rate.[2] Despite promising data, the technique depends heavily on the availability of endoscopic instruments and expertise for mass screening. Therefore, it is key for the efficacious early detection of gastric cancer to perform endoscopy in the high-risk population selected by a promising nonendoscopic biomarker, such as serum pepsinogen status.[3] Furthermore, the introduction of various new endoscopic devices and techniques may enhance the value of endoscopy in efficacious cancer screening. High-definition endoscopy (HDE) and image-enhanced endoscopy,[4] including narrow band imaging (NBI),[5] are the key modalities in advanced endoscopic imaging in gastric cancer.

The authors have nothing to disclose and no conflict of interest.

[a] Department of Gastroenterology, Toranomon Hospital, 2-2-2, Toranomon, Minato-ku, Tokyo 105-8470, Japan

[b] Department of Endoscopy, The Jikei University School of Medicine, 3-25-8 Nishishinbashi, Minato-ku, Tokyo 105-8461, Japan

[c] Department of Gastroenterology and Hepatology, The Jikei University School of Medicine, 3-25-8 Nishishinbashi, Minato-ku, Tokyo 105-8461, Japan

* Corresponding author.

E-mail address: kaise@toranomon.gr.jp

Gastroenterol Clin N Am 39 (2010) 771–784
doi:10.1016/j.gtc.2010.08.028
0889-8553/10/$ – see front matter © 2010 Elsevier Inc. All rights reserved.

HDE IMPROVES THE DETECTION AND DIAGNOSIS OF SUPERFICIAL GASTRIC CANCER

Although upper gastrointestinal (GI) endoscopy is more accurate than nonendoscopic modalities, including integrated positron emission tomography and barium meal examination, it is empirically known that considerable numbers of superficial gastric cancers are missed or misdiagnosed with conventional white light endoscopy (WLE). HDE has been developed for improving the image quality and diagnostic accuracy of WLE. To elucidate the potential of HDE, we prospectively compared ultrathin endoscopy (UTE) with HDE with respect to diagnostic accuracy of superficial gastric neoplasia.[6]

In this study, 32 patients with superficial gastric neoplasia referred for endoscopic submucosal dissection (ESD) were recruited; 25 patients undergoing follow-up endoscopy after ESD were also enrolled as neoplasia-free controls (**Fig. 1**). Patients with obvious advanced gastric carcinomas or cancerous lesions with deep invasion to the gastric submucosa were excluded. Each patient underwent UTE (GIF-XP260N, Olympus Medical Systems Corp, Tokyo, Japan) and HDE (GIF-H260Z, Olympus Medical Systems Corp) back-to-back in a randomized order. UTE and HDE were independently performed by 2 different experienced endoscopists who did not have access to any clinical information before the endoscopic examination. The study coordinator organized the patient data and guided the 2 endoscopists, one at a time, into the endoscopic room. The endoscopists independently performed endoscopic examination under conscious sedation on the same patient and recorded the diagnosis of neoplastic as well as nonneoplastic lesions, including gastric ulcers or gastric polyps. All lesions recorded as neoplastic or nonneoplastic, as well as any neoplastic lesion that was referred for ESD but not detected by either endoscopist, were biopsied by the second endoscopist under the supervision of the study coordinator, who attended all endoscopic examinations and was aware of the diagnosis made by the 2

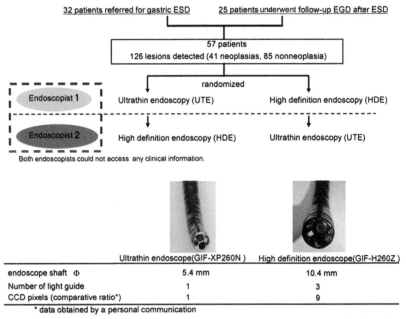

Fig. 1. Study design and the specifications of the ultrathin endoscope and high-definition endoscope used in the study. CCD, charge-coupled device; EGD, esophagogastroduodenoscopy.

endoscopists. The study coordinator could easily notice the existences of gastric neoplasias referred for ESD but missed by the participating endoscopists because he was aware of the pathologic reports and representative endoscopic images recorded at the affiliated hospitals. The pathology results from the biopsy were used as a gold standard for the diagnosis of gastric cancer.

Among 57 enrolled patients, 41 lesions (16.5 ± 13.5 mm in diameter, mean ± SD) were pathologically diagnosed as neoplasias (27 carcinomas and 14 adenomas). Of the 41 pathologically diagnosed neoplasias, 11 were not detected and 3 were diagnosed as nonneoplasias by UTE, indicating that the missing and misdiagnosis rates of UTE were 26.8% and 14.6%, respectively. Similarly, 5 of the 41 pathologically diagnosed neoplasias were not detected and 4 were diagnosed as nonneoplasias by HDE, indicating that the missing and misdiagnosis rates of HDE were 12.2% and 9.8%, respectively. The rate of missed and misdiagnosed proximal lesions (fornix and corpus) was significantly higher for UTE (29%) than for HDE (7.2%) (P = .002). In comparison, the rates of missed lesions and misdiagnosed distal lesions (angulus and antrum) were comparable for UTE and HDE (**Table 1**). Representative neoplastic lesions missed by UTE but correctly diagnosed by HDE are shown in **Fig. 2**.

Although conscious sedation is widely used to reduce endoscopy-induced discomfort and increase acceptance of the procedure, it can cause adverse effects[7] and increases the cost,[8] either directly (medications, additional time required to sedate and recover the patients) or indirectly (time lost from work by both the patient and the patient's escort). UTE has emerged as an alternative to sedated conventional upper GI endoscopy for screening because it is well tolerated in the absence of sedation and is less costly.[9] However, the authors' study demonstrated that the diagnostic accuracy of HDE is significantly higher than that of UTE for superficial gastric neoplasia and that this difference is particularly striking for neoplasias in the proximal stomach. We need to adequately select HDE or UTE in different clinical settings by recognizing the differences in the diagnostic accuracy and the acceptance without sedation.

THE CLINICAL VALUE OF AUTOFLUORESCENCE ENDOSCOPY IS LIMITED IN GASTRIC CANCER

Although HDE improves the diagnostic accuracy of WLE, more than 20% of superficial gastric neoplasias are still missed or misdiagnosed. Image-enhanced endoscopy,

Table 1
Comparison of the diagnostic accuracy of UTE and HDE in the diagnosis of gastric cancer

(A) Comparison of the diagnostic accuracy in the diagnosis of gastric cancer

	Sensitivity		Specificity	
UTE	58.5%	P = 0.021	91.8%	P = 0.014
HDE	78.0%		100%	

(B) Rates of missed and misdiagnosed lesions including neoplasia and nonneoplasia

	All Lesions (95% CI[a])		Distal Lesions (Angulus-Antrum)		Proximal Lesions (Fornix-Corpus)	
UTE	27.1% (18.5–38.3%)	P<0.001	24.5% (13.3–38.9%)	P = 0.19	29.0% (18.7–41.1%)	P = 0.002
HDE	9.3% (4.7–16.7%)		12.2% (4.6–24.7%)		7.2% (2.4–16.1%)	

Abbreviations: HDE, high definition endoscopy; UTE, ultrathin endoscopy.
[a] 95% CI: 95% confidential Interval.

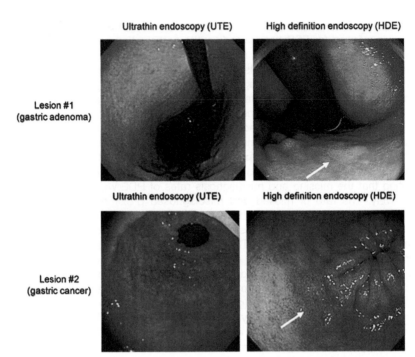

Fig. 2. Representative endoscopic images of 2 neoplastic lesions missed by UTE but correctly diagnosed by HDE. Lesion No.1 located in the upper gastric corpus is a white superficial elevation that was pathologically diagnosed as gastric adenoma. Lesion No. 2 located in the antrum is a superficial depression that was resected by ESD and diagnosed pathologically as mucosal cancer. (*From* Toyoizumi H, Kaise M, Arakawa H, et al. Ultrathin endoscopy vs high-resolution endoscopy for diagnosing superficial gastric neoplasia: a prospective comparative study. Gastrointest Endosc 2009;70(2):243; with permission.)

including autofluorescence endoscopy (AFE) and NBI, has been developed for overcoming the limit of WLE. There has been considerable interest in the use of AFE for the detection of early neoplasias, and the diagnostic relevance of the modality has been demonstrated for the detection of early neoplasias in the esophagus[10] and colon.[11,12]

Therefore, the authors conducted a prospective study to systematically compare AFE with WLE for the detection of superficial gastric neoplasia.[13] The authors enrolled an enriched population of 33 patients with superficial gastric neoplasia referred for ESD and 18 patients undergoing follow-up endoscopy after curative ESD as control. An autofluorescence imaging system (CLV-260SL and CV-260 SL, Olympus Medical Systems Corp) and the autofluorescence imaging scope (XGIF-Q240FZ, Olympus Medical Systems) were used for the AFE procedure. The new autofluorescence system enables selection of either a red-green-blue illumination for normal WLE or an excitation/reflected light combination for AFE. At the direction of a study coordinator, 2 endoscopists blinded to the patient's history and to each other's findings, performed WLE followed by AFE or AFE alone, in a random order. Both endoscopists independently recorded the presence of lesions observed by AFE and WLE. All lesions identified in either test were biopsied, and the pathologic results were used as the gold standard.

A total of 39 gastric neoplasias were histologically confirmed, and 52 pathologically diagnosed nonneoplastic lesions were found to be either WLE- and/or AFE-positive. Sensitivities of WLE and AFE alone were 74% and 64% (*P* = .79), respectively, and specificities of WLE and AFE alone were 83% and 40% (*P* = .0003), respectively. WLE followed by AFE had a sensitivity of 69% (nonsignificant) and a specificity of 64% (*P* = .046) compared with WLE alone. AFE detected 13% of all neoplasias finally diagnosed (23% of elevated neoplasias), which were missed by WLE.

Although one-quarter of elevated gastric neoplasias were detected only by AFE, it was concluded that its specificity is poor because of the high rate of false-positive detection of lesions, such as intestinal metaplasia or regenerative hyperplasia; therefore the clinical value of AFE is limited. **Fig. 3** shows false-positive detection of lesions by AFE, and **Fig. 4** demonstrates a representative gastric cancer that was missed by WLE but detected by AFE in the prospective study.

DIAGNOSTIC CRITERIA FOR GASTRIC CANCER USING MAGNIFYING ENDOSCOPY COMBINED WITH NBI

NBI[5] is an innovative optical technology that modifies the wave lengths and bandwidths of an endoscope's light into narrow band illumination of 415 ± 30 nm and 540 ± 30 nm (**Fig. 5**). By using these narrow spectrums that fall within the hemoglobin absorption band and penetrate only into the superficial depth of the mucosa, NBI markedly improves the contrast of vascular structures and, combined with magnifying endoscopy (ME), yields clearer images of microvasculature and fine mucosal structure (FMS) in the GI tract. ME combined with NBI (ME-NBI) may enable endoscopic diagnoses based on cancer-specific alterations in the FMS or microvasculature and can

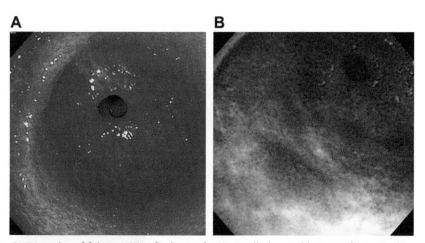

A   **B**

Fig. 3. Examples of false-positive findings of AFE. Small elevated lesions of intestinal metaplasia or regenerative hyperplasia in atrophic gastric mucosa appeared as highly positive findings at AFE, that is, as magenta surrounded by green. Multiple erosions are identified by WLE (*A*). AFE shows nonneoplastic erosions as a magenta lesion with a defined circumferential margin within green mucosa, which is regarded as a positive finding at AFE (*B*). The lesion was pathologically proven to be nonneoplastic. (*From* Kato M, Kaise M, Yonezawa J, et al. Autofluorescence endoscopy vs conventional white light endoscopy for the detection of superficial gastric neoplasia: a prospective comparative study. Endoscopy 2007;39(11):940; with permission.)

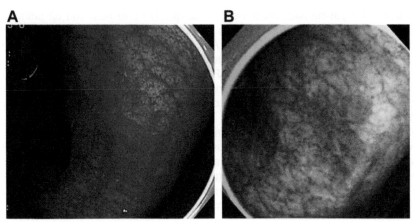

Fig. 4. An example of superficial gastric neoplasia detected by AFE but missed by WLE. WLE did not detect this notable lesion in the atrophic corpus mucosa (A). AFE shows a magenta lesion within green mucosa, deemed therefore to be AFE-positive (B). The lesion was resected by ESD and pathologically proved to be a gastric cancer in adenoma. (*From* Kato M, Kaise M, Yonezawa J, et al. Autofluorescence endoscopy vs conventional white light endoscopy for the detection of superficial gastric neoplasia: a prospective comparative study. Endoscopy 2007;39(11):940; with permission.)

achieve "endoscopic pathology," whereby an accurate endoscopic diagnosis comparable with a histopathologic diagnosis can be made without biopsy sampling. Thus, the authors have performed a study to elucidate the cancer-specific microstructural findings obtained with ME-NBI and define the criteria for gastric cancer diagnosis with ME-NBI.[14]

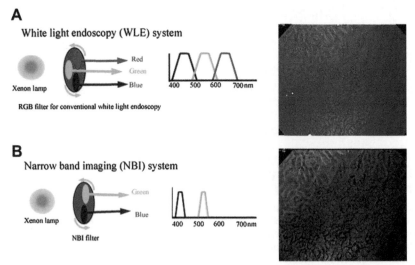

Fig. 5. Differences between WLE (A) and NBI systems (B). The NBI filter consists of 2 narrow bands (415 ± 30 nm and 540 ± 30 nm, respectively) that yield a clearer image of the microvasculature and fine mucosal structures in the gastric mucosa and superficial gastric cancer than that obtained by WLE. RGB, red-green-blue.

First, an ME-NBI catalog composed of 100 lesions (55 depressed gastric cancers and 45 noncancerous depressions) was constructed. On reviewing the catalog without access to the clinical and pathologic data, 11 endoscopists answered as to the presence or absence of predefined microstructural findings obtained with ME-NBI (**Fig. 6**). These findings consisted of microvascular features (dilation, denseness, tortuousness, regionality, abrupt caliber alteration, and heterogeneity in shape) and features of the FMS (absence or unclearness, micrification, and heterogeneity in shape).

Multivariate logistic regression analysis demonstrated significant associations between gastric cancer and 5 ME-NBI findings (**Table 2**). Among the microvascular features, dilation, tortuousness, abrupt caliber alteration, and heterogeneity in shape were significantly linked with gastric cancer. Among the FMS features, only absence or unclearness was significantly linked with gastric cancer. Diagnostic figures to model the probability of the presence of gastric cancer detected by ME-NBI were compared by the area under the curve (AUC) of the receiver operating characteristic curves. The AUC for all ME-NBI features was 0.864 (95% confidence interval [CI], 0.840–0.887). To identify a minimal diagnostic criterion that would maintain superior diagnostic accuracy while combining as few as possible of the 9 predefined features, the authors compared the AUC for all ME-NBI features with that for various combinations of microstructural abnormalities. The triad of FMS disappearance, microvascular dilation, and heterogeneity was the smallest combination that had an AUC of 0.848 (95% CI, 0.825–0.870), comparable to the AUC of all ME-NBI features (**Fig. 7**). According to the data, this triad (FMS disappearance, microvascular dilation, and heterogeneity)

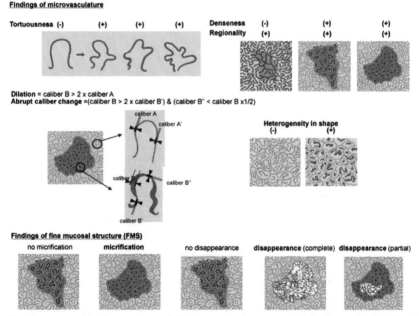

Fig. 6. Scheme used to demonstrate definitions of microstructural findings obtained by ME-NBI. (*From* Kaise M, Kato M, Urashima M, et al. Magnifying endoscopy combined with narrow-band imaging for differential diagnosis of superficial depressed gastric lesions. Endoscopy 2009;41(4):312; with permission.)

Table 2
Multivariate logistic regression analysis on the associations between defined ME-NBI findings and superficial depressed gastric cancer

	Findings	Odds Ratio	95% CI	P Value
Microvasculature	Dilation	1.89	1 27–2.78	.001
	Tortuousness	1.88	1.23–2.37	.004
	Heterogeneity	1.95	[1.16–3.24]	.009
	Abrupt caliber alteration	1.86	[1.19–2.39]	.006
	Denseness	0.73	[0.50–1.06]	.100
	Regionality	0.75	[0.44–1.28]	.290
FMS	Disappearance	5.47	[3.72–8.05]	>.001
	Micrification	1.07	[0.72–1.59]	.74
	Heterogeneity	1.02	[0.68–1.53]	.68

Abbreviation: CI, confidence interval.

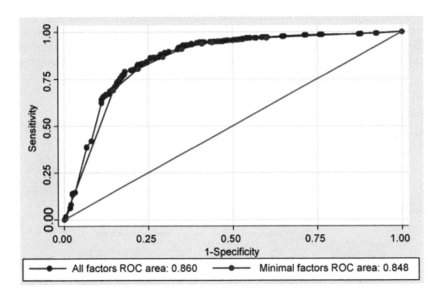

The minimal factors (The triad)	Odds ratio	[95% C I]	P value
microvascular dilation	2.52	[1.80 – 3.53]	> .001
microvascular heterogeneity	4.44	[3.13 – 6.31]	> .001
FMS disappearance	5.98	[4.14 – 8.64]	> .001

Fig. 7. The graph demonstrates receiver operating characteristic (ROC) curves to model the probability of the presence of gastric cancer from ME-NBI findings. The blue line is the ROC curve with all ME-NBI findings, and the red line is the ROC curve with the triad used for the minimal ME-NBI criterion. Areas under the 2 ROC curves are comparable. (*From* Kaise M, Kato M, Urashima M, et al. Magnifying endoscopy combined with narrow-band imaging for differential diagnosis of superficial depressed gastric lesions. Endoscopy 2009; 41(4):313; with permission.)

has been adopted as the minimal criterion for gastric cancer diagnosis with ME-NBI (**Fig. 8**).

Representative WLE, indigo carmine chromoendoscopy, and ME-NBI images of gastric cancer and noncancerous depression are shown in **Fig. 9**.

ME-NBI ACHIEVES SUPERIOR ACCURACY IN DIFFERENTIAL DIAGNOSIS OF GASTRIC CANCER—A PROSPECTIVE STUDY

Next, a prospective study was performed to elucidate the superiority of ME-NBI over WLE in gastric cancer diagnosis using the minimal criterion (the triad).[15] To scientifically compare the diagnostic accuracy of WLE and ME-NBI, each modality should be separately and independently performed for excluding carryover effects of the other modality of comparison. However, ME-NBI is not suitable for examining the whole stomach because of the weak light intensity of NBI and is clinically used as a technique to further characterize lesions in the stomach detected by WLE. Therefore, the authors performed a prospective study to evaluate the superiority of ME-NBI in the differential diagnosis of superficial gastric lesions identified with conventional WLE.

A total of 111 patients who underwent WLE and ME-NBI for surveying synchronous or metachronous cancer because of having a high risk of gastric cancer were recruited (**Fig. 10**). WLE without using magnification was performed first, and superficial gastric lesions were included as follows: 79 lesions that were diagnosed by WLE as cancerous and 122 lesions that were diagnosed by WLE as noncancerous but required pathologic evaluation because of having a slight suspicion of cancer. ME-NBI and biopsy were done sequentially for all lesions included for evaluation. Diagnoses of cancer by ME-NBI were made either on the basis of each endoscopist's impression of the lesion (personal diagnosis) or using the diagnostic triad detailed later (triad-based diagnosis). Pathologic diagnoses of biopsied samples were used as the gold standard for cancer diagnosis.

A total of 201 lesions (mean diameter 7.0 ± 4.0 mm) from 111 patients (98 men and 13 women; mean age 66.3 years) were evaluated. Of the 201 lesions, 14 were pathologically proved to be cancerous and the others were noncancerous lesions

Minimal criteria (the triad) for gastric cancer diagnosis with magnifying endoscopy combined with NBI (ME-NBI)

1) Disappearance or unclearness of fine mucosal structure (FMS)

2) Vascular dilation

3) Vascular heterogeneity

Disappearance of fine mucosal structure

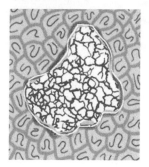 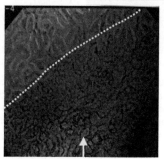

Vascular dilation and heterogeneity in shape

Fig. 8. Scheme and representative image of minimal criterion (the triad) for gastric cancer diagnosis with ME-NBI.

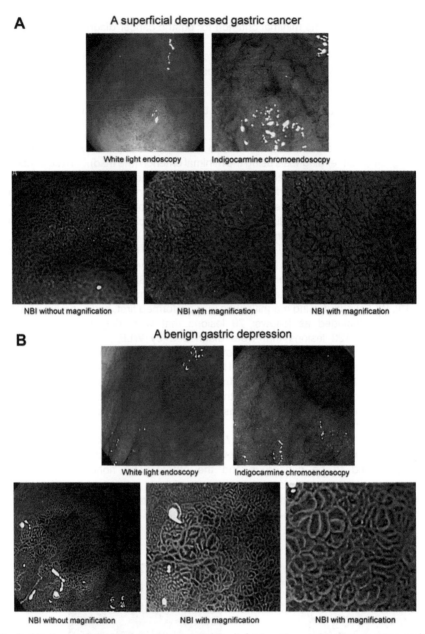

Fig. 9. (*A*) A superficial depressed cancer. White light imaging and indigo carmine endoscopy show a small depression, but it is hard to diagnose as gastric cancer. ME-NBI shows the existence of the minimal criterion (the triad: disappearance of the FMS, vascular dilation, and heterogeneity in shape), and the lesion can be diagnosed as cancer. The lesion was resected with ESD and was pathologically proven as well differentiated adenocarcinoma. (*B*) A superficial noncancerous depression. White light imaging and indigo carmine endoscopy show a small depression, but it is hard to diagnose gastric cancer or benign lesion. ME-NBI shows the existence of FMS and no vascular dilation and heterogeneity in shape, indicating that the lesion is not cancerous but benign. The pathology of biopsy specimens showed no cancerous change but regenerative atypia.

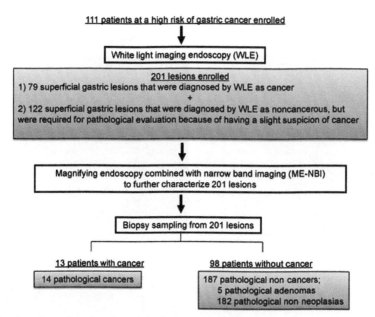

Fig. 10. Flow chart showing the study design and results.

(5 adenomas and 182 nonneoplastic lesions); 79 of the 201 superficial gastric lesions were recognized or suspected as cancerous lesions with WLE. However, only 6 of these 79 lesions (7.6%) were determined to be cancerous pathologically. Of the 79 lesions, 13% were diagnosed as cancerous by NBI. The remaining 87% of lesions diagnosed as cancerous by WLE were diagnosed as noncancerous by NBI, and all but 1 lesion detected as cancerous by WLE and 1 detected as noncancerous by NBI were determined to be cancerous pathologically. The sensitivity and specificity for ME-NBI diagnosis using the triad (92.9% and 94.7%, respectively) were significantly better than those for WLE (42.9% and 61.0%, respectively; P<.0001) (**Table 3**).

Fig. 11 shows 2 representative lesions included in this study: (1) a pathologically noncancerous depression that was diagnosed by WLE as cancerous but by ME-NBI as noncancerous and (2) a pathologically cancerous depression that was diagnosed by WLE as noncancerous but by ME-NBI as cancerous.

FUTURE PERSPECTIVE OF NBI IN GASTRIC CANCER

ME-NBI achieved superior accuracy in the differential diagnosis of superficial gastric lesions identified by WLE. Thus, ME-NBI may increase the diagnostic value of

Table 3		
Comparison of the diagnostic accuracy of WLE and ME-NBI in the diagnosis of gastric cancer		
	Sensitivity (95% CI)	**Specificity (95% CI)**
WLE General Diagnosis	42.9 (35.9–49.6)[a]	61.0 (54.5–67.9)[b]
ME-NBI Personal Diagnosis	85.7 (80.7–90.4)[b]	90.9 (87.1–95.0)[b]
ME-NBI Diagnosis With the Triad	92.9 (89.5–96.6)[b]	94.7 (91.4–97.7)[b]

[a] P<.05.
[b] P<.0001.

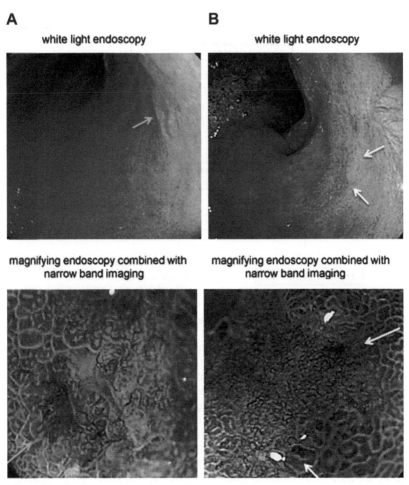

Fig. 11. The lesion shown in (*A*) was a pathologically diagnosed adenocarcinoma that was diagnosed by WLE as noncancerous with a slight suspicion of cancer but by ME-NBI as cancerous because the findings met the minimal criterion of the triad: disappearance of the FMS, microvascular dilation, and heterogeneity. Blue arrows indicate the same position of the lesion in the images of WLE and ME-NBI. The lesion shown in (*B*) was a pathologically diagnosed cancerous lesion that was diagnosed by WLE as noncancerous but by ME-NBI as cancerous because the findings met the minimal criterion. White and yellow arrows indicate the same positions of the lesion in the images of WLE and ME-NBI, respectively.

endoscopy in a population at a high risk of gastric cancer. ME-NBI may reduce unnecessary oversampling of noncancerous gastric lesions for subsequent pathologic differentiation, thus decreasing the costs associated with the diagnosis of gastric cancer. Several endoscopic modalities have been developed or are currently being developed to achieve endoscopic pathology, resulting in a more accurate endoscopic diagnosis that is comparable to a histopathologic diagnosis. Endocytoscopy, a contact ultrahigh ME, can display endoscopic images at 1000 times magnification, making atypical cells and structures visible.[16] Similarly, confocal laser microendoscopy yields diagnostic images comparable with histopathologic findings.[17] These modalities classified as endoscopic microscopy are attractive because they can be used to discover histologic alterations of the mucosal layer at cellular and subcellular resolution. However, these techniques require intravenous or endoluminal administration of a dye or fluorescent reagent, which limits their clinical use. In contrast, NBI enhances the quality of microstructure imaging without the need of a dye or fluorescent staining and thus may be a promising modality for endoscopic pathology in a standard clinical setting. The light intensity of NBI is so weak that it is hard to observe the whole stomach only with NBI, and NBI is generally used in combination with ME to further characterize lesions detected by WLE, especially in the stomach. In contrast to the stomach, NBI achieved higher detection rates than WLE in the esophagus and pharynx.[18] Future innovation on the light intensity and NBI system may overcome the limitation and increase its detection ability without WLE, even in the stomach.

REFERENCES

1. Ma X, Yu H. Global burden of cancer. Yale J Biol Med 2006;79:85–94.
2. Tashiro A, Sano M, Kinameri K, et al. Comparing mass screening techniques for gastric cancer in Japan. World J Gastroenterol 2006;12:4874–5.
3. Watabe H, Mitsushima T, Yamaji Y, et al. Predicting the development of gastric cancer from combining *Helicobacter pylori* antibodies and serum pepsinogen status: a prospective endoscopic cohort study. Gut 2005;54:764–8.
4. Tajiri H, Niwa H. Proposal for a consensus terminology in endoscopy: how should different endoscopic imaging techniques be grouped and defined? Endoscopy 2008;40:775–8.
5. Gono K, Yamazaki K, Doguchi N, et al. Endoscopic observation of tissue by narrow band illumination. Opt Rev 2003;10:211–5.
6. Toyoizumi H, Kaise M, Arakawa H, et al. Ultrathin endoscopy versus high-resolution endoscopy for diagnosing superficial gastric neoplasia: a prospective comparative study. Gastrointest Endosc 2009;70:240–5.
7. Froehlich F, Schwizer W, Thorens J, et al. Conscious sedation for gastroscopy: patient tolerance and cardiorespiratory parameters. Gastroenterology 1995; 108:697–704.
8. Mokhashi MS, Hawes RH. Struggling towards easier endoscopy. Gastrointest Endosc 1998;48:432–40.
9. Garcia RT, Cello JP, Nguyen MH, et al. Unsedated ultrathin EGD is well accepted when compared with conventional sedated EGD: a multicenter randomized trial. Gastroenterology 2003;125:1606–12.
10. Kara MA, Peters FP, ten Kate FJW, et al. Endoscopic video autofluorescence imaging may improve the detection of early neoplasia in patients with Barrett's esophagus. Gastrointest Endosc 2005;61:679–85.
11. McCallum AL, Jenkins JT, Gillen D, et al. Evaluation of autofluorescence colonoscopy for the detection and diagnosis of colonic polyps. Gastrointest Endosc 2008;68:283–90.
12. Aihara H, Sumiyama K, Saito S, et al. Numerical analysis of the autofluorescence intensity of neoplastic and non-neoplastic colorectal lesions by using a novel videoendoscopy system. Gastrointest Endosc 2009;69:726–33.
13. Kato M, Kaise M, Yonezawa J, et al. Autofluorescence endoscopy versus conventional white light endoscopy for the detection of superficial gastric neoplasia; a prospective comparative study. Endoscopy 2007;39:937–41.
14. Kaise M, Kato M, Arakawa H, et al. Magnifying endoscopy combined with narrow-band imaging for differential diagnosis of superficial depressed gastric lesions. Endoscopy 2009;41:310–5.

15. Kato M, Kaise M, Yonezawa J, et al. Magnifying endoscopy with narrow band imaging achieves superior accuracy in the differential diagnosis of superficial gastric lesions identified with white light endoscopy: a prospective study. Gastrointest Endosc 2010;72(3):523–9.
16. Inoue H, Kudo S, Shiokawa A. Novel endoscopic imaging techniques toward in vivo observation of living cancer cells in the gastrointestinal tract. Clin Gastroenterol Hepatol 2005;3:61–3.
17. Kiesslich R, Burg J, Vieth M, et al. Confocal laser endoscopy for diagnosing intraepithelial neoplasias and colorectal cancer in vivo. Gastroenterology 2004;127: 706–13.
18. Muto M, Katada K, Omori T, et al. Early detection of superficial squamous cell carcinoma in the head and neck region and esophagus by narrow band imaging: a multicenter randomized controlled trial. J Clin Oncol 2010;28:1566–72.

Endomicroscopy of Intestinal Metaplasia and Gastric Cancer

Chang-Qing Li, MD, PhD, Yan-Qing Li, MD, PhD*

KEYWORDS

• Endomicroscopy • Intestinal metaplasia • Gastric cancer

Gastric intestinal metaplasia (GIM) is regarded as a precancerous lesion with the risk of developing into intestinal-type gastric cancer (GC)[1]; hence, endoscopic diagnosis of GIM is valuable for patients undergoing surveillance endoscopy.[2] Biopsy is normally required to confirm the diagnosis of GIM because diagnosis of GIM by using conventional endoscopy is unreliable.[3–5]

On the other hand, endoscopy is the current touchstone of GC diagnosis. With the development of endoscopy, endoscopists nowadays can predict not only the malignancy of a lesion but also its histologic phenotype.[6] During the evolution of endoscopic diagnosis, knowledge and technology are inseparable. There is no doubt that as technology advances, endoscopists could give real-time histologic diagnosis.

Confocal laser endomicroscopy (CLE), with its optical biopsy utility aided by fluorescein contrast agents and the most significant magnification power at present,[7–9] assists in the in vivo histologic diagnosis of GIM and GC.[10–14] The aim of this review is to describe the endomicroscopic features of GIM and GC and review their clinical applications.

STAINING AGENTS IN CLE
Fluorescein Sodium

Fluorescein sodium is the most common contrast agent used in CLE,[15] and intravenous fluorescein sodium alone is sufficient in the diagnosis of GIM. In the diagnosis of GC, tissue structure and microvessels could be well displayed by using fluorescein sodium. Although the outline of each cell is identifiable with fluorescein sodium, the intracellular architecture, particularly the nuclei, could not be displayed.[16]

In the allergy test before the procedure, 1 mL of 2% fluorescein sodium should be given. For observation with CLE, another standard 5 mL of 10% fluorescein sodium is intravenously injected. Severe complications were not reported so far. Mild allergic

The authors have nothing to disclose.
Department of Gastroenterology, Shandong University Qilu Hospital, No 107, Wenhuaxi Road, Jinan 250012, China
* Corresponding author.
E-mail address: liyanqing@sdu.edu.cn

0889-8553/10/$ – see front matter © 2010 Elsevier Inc. All rights reserved.

reactions including pruritus and rash are rare and can be overcome by temporary anti-allergic treatment. The most common side effects, yellow-stained skin and urine, usually resolve in 24 hours.[7,17]

Acriflavine

With specific binding to DNA, topical acriflavine stains nuclei specifically under CLE. The most frequently applied concentration of acriflavine is 0.02%.[18] Too high concentration of acriflavine stains the whole cell, which makes nuclei unidentifiable, and too low concentration decreases image quality.

Although this agent was reported as having risks of carcinogenesis in animal experiments, evidence is still lacking for human beings.[18]

Cresyl Violet

Cresyl violet is another common staining agent that negatively stains the nuclei in CLE image. However, current evidence supports its application only in the colon and small intestine.[19] Evidence of its application in stomach is not yet available.

GIM
Microscopy of GIM

The conventional diagnosis of GIM still depends on biopsy and histology, although advanced white light endoscopy could predict the histologic diagnosis more accurately than conventional endoscopy.[3,5,20–22] The histologic characterization of GIM is essential for its in vivo CLE diagnosis.

The present classification of GIM consists of type I (complete) and types II and III (incomplete). Type I (complete GIM) appears similar to the normal small intestinal mucosa, with goblet cells and absorptive cells arranged beneath a brush border. In incomplete GIM, the typical enterocytes are replaced by intermediate cells lacking a well-developed brush border. Type II shows glandular distortion and consists of goblet cells and columnar mucous cells secreting sialomucins. Type III is characterized by glandular distortion and columnar mucous cells containing sulfomucins.[23]

Type III is associated with higher risks of development into intestinal-type GC.[24,25] Although some investigators suggested that the predictive value of GIM types be limited,[26] others recommended that patients with type III GIM be closely followed up.[2] Therefore, the diagnosis of GIM involves both identification and classification.

Endoscopy of GIM

There are no standard endoscopic features that distinguish GIM from the normal mucosa. Detection of GIM by using conventional endoscopy relies on random biopsy and histology. At present, the in vivo endoscopic identification of GIM is achieved only by using some advanced endoscopic technologies, such as chromoendoscopy, magnification endoscopy, narrow band imaging (NBI), and enhanced magnification endoscopy, alone or in combination.[3,27–30] The endoscopic features of GIM are based on the assessment of gastric pit patterns and color changes.

The observation by Guelrud and colleagues[27] using enhanced magnification endoscopy reveals 4 patterns of the gastric mucosa: (1) round pits, a characteristic pit pattern of regular and orderly arranged circular dots; (2) reticular, pits that are circular or oval and regular in shape and arrangement; (3) villous, no pits present but a fine villiform appearance, with the villi having a regular shape and arrangement; and (4) ridged, no pits present but cerebriform with regular shape and arrangement of the villi. The results of their observation suggest that type III and type IV correlate with the histologic identification of GIM.[27] Although the sensitivity of enhanced magnification endoscopy for detection of GIM was good (94%), the specificity was poor (64%). The classification system was not applied to differentiate complete from incomplete GIM. In addition, the intraobserver and interobserver variabilities were not evaluated.

Some investigators suggested the combination of chromoendoscopy and magnification endoscopy to be applied in both identification and classification of GIM. Dinis-Ribeiro and colleagues[3] classified the gastric mucosa into 3 groups based on 2 variables: pit patterns and change in color of the mucosa after application of methylene blue. Group I is defined as having regular pit pattern and no color change, which represents nonmetaplastic nondysplastic mucosa. Group II is defined as having regular pit pattern and blue color change, which represents GIM. Group III is defined as having neither a clear pit pattern nor a clear color change, which represents dysplastic mucosa. Group II is divided into 4 subgroups according to detailed pit patterns as follows: blue irregular marks (IIA), blue round and tubular pits (IIB), blue villi (IIC), and blue small pits (IID). The study revealed that IIA and IIB were more often associated with complete GIM and IIC and IID with incomplete GIM. For the diagnosis of GIM, this classification had an accuracy of 82%, a sensitivity of 76%, and a specificity of 87%. The overall accuracy of the diagnosis of complete and incomplete GIM was 84% and 82%, respectively. In reproducibility assessment, although interobserver and intraobserver agreements were substantial for classification by groups, the agreements were only moderate for classification by subgroups, such as types IIA to IID. Therefore, the diagnostic criteria are reliable for identification of GIM, but the classification of GIM based on them needs to be confirmed.

NBI is a novel endoscopic technology that is based on the principle of modifying the spectral characteristics of the illuminating light by narrowing the bandwidth of the optical filter in the light source. Some studies showed that the appearance of a light blue crest (LBC) in the mucosa is a distinctive endoscopic finding, suggesting an increased likelihood of detecting GIM. The LBC appears as bluish white patchy areas in NBI. Uedo and colleagues[28] reported that identification of LBC had a sensitivity of 89%, a specificity of 93%, and an accuracy of 91% for the diagnosis of GIM. It was speculated that the appearance of the LBC was caused by the difference in the reflectance of the light at the surface of the ciliated tissue structure. Whether LBC could be applied in the classification of GIM was not reported, and the interobserver or intraobserver variability needs further evaluation.

In summary, the current endoscopic diagnosis of GIM relies on indirect characteristics such as pit patterns and color change (by staining agents or optical methods). These characteristics increase the accuracy of in vivo diagnosis of GIM. However, the direct evidences of GIM, such as presence of goblet cells, could not be obtained, and classification of GIM phenotypes by these technologies is still difficult.[27,28] Although the combination of chromoendoscopy and magnification endoscopy could differentiate complete from incomplete GIM, with moderate interobserver agreement,[3] the preparation and process of chromoendoscopy are complicated and time consuming. Furthermore, a recent report suggested that methylene blue chromoendoscopy induced questionable oxidative DNA damage.[31]

Endomicroscopy of GIM

As a combination of endoscopy and in vivo microscopy, endomicroscopy should serve in the real-time identification and classification of GIM.

Identification of GIM by endomicroscopy

The endomicroscopic identification of GIM is based on both histology and endoscopy, the latter depends mostly on evaluation of gastric pit patterns.[3,20] Therefore, the criteria for CLE diagnosis of gastric lesions, including GIM, begin with the classification of gastric pit patterns. According to the study by Zhang and colleagues[10], the gastric pit patterns are classified into 7 types:

Type A; round pits with round openings, representing normal mucosal with fundic glands.

Type B; noncontinuous, short, rodlike pits with short threadlike openings, representing corporal mucosa with chronic inflammation.

Type C is continuous, short, rodlike pits with slitlike opening, representing normal mucosa with pyloric glands.

Type D is elongated, tortuous, branchlike pits representing antral mucosa with chronic inflammation.

Type E is decreased number of prominently dilated pits representing chronic atrophy gastritis.

Type F represents GIM and has villuslike appearance, an interstitium in the center, and goblet cells.

Type G represents GC with normal pits disappearing, with appearance of atypical cells or glands.

Guo and colleagues[11] refined the CLE imaging of GIM into 3 features: goblet cells, columnar absorptive cells and brush border, and villiform foveolar epithelium. GIM was determined if any of the 3 features were present. The diagnosis based on the 3 features has a sensitivity of 98.13% and a specificity of 95.33%. The kappa score for the correlation between CLE and histopathology was 0.94. Details of the 3 GIM features are as follows:

- Goblet cells: large black cells with mucin
- Columnar absorptive cells and brush border: more slender and brighter than columnar mucous cells of normal gastric mucosa, with a clear dark line at the surface of the epithelium
- Villiform foveolar epithelium: a typical villouslike appearance different from the antral or corpus foveolae gastricae.

Among the 3 features, presence of goblet cells seems to be the most sensitive marker of GIM under CLE.[32] Presence of goblet cells is also the well-established hallmark of GIM in conventional histology, because they are absent in normal gastric musoca.[23] Bao and colleagues[33] used two-photon fluorescence endomicroscopy to examine the mouse intestine, which has goblet cells, as a model of intestinal metaplasia. One-photon confocal fluorescence endomicroscopy and two-photon fluorescence endomicroscopy were used for 3-dimensional imaging of goblet cells. Both the techniques can 3-dimensionally view goblet cells in mouse large intestine and achieve an imaging depth of 176 μm.

Although with significant features, diagnosis of GIM by using CLE is still limited by the penetration depth, which is 250 μm at most. GIM in deeper layers of the mucosa could be missed by current CLE techniques.[34]

Classification of GIM by endomicroscopy

In the study by Guo and colleagues,[11] GIMs were classified as complete (type I) and incomplete (type II or type III) based on morphology and mucin staining with alcian blue (AB) with or without periodic acid–Schiff and high-iron diamine with or without AB, the mucin staining being applied in parallel sections for this purpose.

In the CLE images, GIM was also further classified as complete or incomplete based on the shape of goblet cells, the presence of absorptive cells or brush border, and the architecture of vessels and crypts as follows:

- Complete: goblet cells interspersed among absorptive cells with or without brush borders; with regular crypts and capillaries
- Incomplete: smaller numbers of goblet cells scattered among gastric type cells (mucous cells); without absorptive cells and brush border; with tortuous and branched crypts or irregular capillaries.

The sensitivity, specificity, positive predictive value, and negative predictive value of CLE for the diagnosis of complete GIM was 68.03%, 89.66%, 84.69%, and 76.92%, respectively, and those of incomplete GIM was 68.42%, 83.41%, 40.63%, and 94.09%, respectively. The kappa score for the agreement between CLE and histopathology was 0.67.[11] **Fig. 1** shows the CLE images of the subtypes of GIM and their corresponding histologic features.

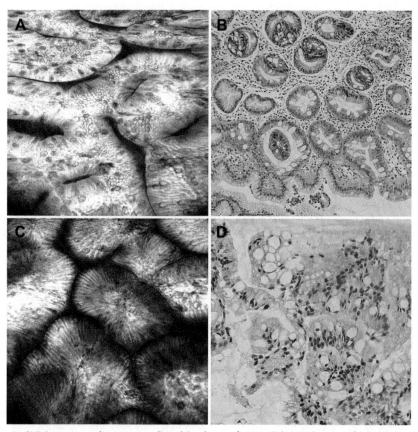

Fig. 1. CLE images and corresponding histology of GIM. (*A*) CLE image of complete GIM shows the villouslike foveolar epithelium with goblet cells and absorptive cells. (*B*) Corresponding histologic image of complete GIM with regular glands, goblet cells, and columnar mucous cells (hematoxylin-eosin [HE], ×200). (*C*) CLE image of incomplete GIM shows tortuous foveolae with smaller numbers of goblet cells than complete GIM. (*D*) Corresponding histologic image of incomplete GIM. Small and less numerous goblet cell vacuoles with irregular glands can be seen (HE, ×400).

GC
Microscopy of GC

Several histologic classifications of GC, such as the World Health Organization, Ming, Lauren, Nakamura, and Goseki classifications, have been proposed. The Lauren classification presented in 1965 was widely accepted. This classification has advantages in that it distinguishes, by microscopic morphology alone, 2 main cancer pathogeneses that have clearly dissimilar clinical and epidemiologic entities (diffuse and intestinal subtypes).[35] The intestinal-type GC is conventionally regarded as the well-differentiated type, and the diffuse-type GC as the poorly differentiated type. In general, intestinal-type tumors have a glandular pattern accompanied by papillary structure or dense components. The glandular pseudostratified epithelium consists of large pleomorphic cells with increased nuclear to cytoplasmic ratio. The polarization of columnar cells is usually preserved. On the contrary, diffuse-type GC is predominantly composed of atypical cells, without any forms of gland.[23]

Similar to the diagnosis of GIM mentioned earlier, the diagnosis of GC by using CLE also includes identification and classification.

Endoscopy of GC

Because advanced GC is easily detected by using conventional endoscopy, the focus of endoscopic diagnosis of GC is on the detection of early GC (EGC). Advanced endoscopy for diagnosis of EGC also includes chromoendoscopy, magnification endoscopy, enhanced magnification endoscopy, and NBI.[6,36–43] Given the complicated and time-consuming process of chromoendoscopy, combining it with conventional endoscopy is not practical for the in vivo diagnosis of EGC. Chromoendoscopy alone is still used only for detection of suspected lesions, whereas chromoendoscopy in combination with magnification endoscopy is generally required for further identification and classification of EGC. Some investigators suggested that the fine surface pattern of gastric carcinomas is often too subtle to be detected with a standard magnification endoscope, and adherent mucus or excessive dye makes magnification chromoendoscopy of the stomach difficult.[39] So most of the recent studies were focused on magnification combined with NBI and enhanced magnification endoscopy. The endoscopic diagnosis is mainly based on assessment of surface pattern and microvascular alterations.

Tanaka and colleagues[39] classified the surface pattern of gastric mucosa into 5 types by using enhanced magnification endoscopy:

Type I, small round pits of uniform size and shape
Type II, slitlike pits
Type III, gyrus and villous patterns
Type IV, irregular arrangements and sizes of pattern types
Type V, destructive patterns.

In a pilot study involving 47 patients with EGC or adenoma, the investigators found that types IV and V were more associated with EGC. To evaluate the efficacy of the classification for identifying EGC, they conducted conventional magnification endoscopy, magnification chromoendoscopy, and enhanced magnification endoscopy on 380 consecutive patients. The results showed that enhanced magnification endoscopy was significantly superior to conventional magnification endoscopy and magnification chromoendoscopy in detection of EGC. Classification of types IV and V strongly correlated with the presence of GC (sensitivity 100%, specificity 89.7%).

However, the positive predictive value was only 40%, which indicates that biopsy accuracy needs to be improved.[6]

Endoscopic assessment of microvessels in EGC by using magnification endoscopy combined with NBI has been studied. A quantitative assessment of the microvessels in gastric mucosa was conducted by using magnification combined with NBI. The mean calibers of microvessels in both differentiated and undifferentiated GC were significantly greater than that in the surrounding mucosa. The mean caliber of microvessels in differentiated GC was greater than that in undifferentiated GC but without significant difference. However, the high failure rate of good-quality image acquisition made almost half of the patients unsuitable for analysis (61/132).[37] Except for assessment of microvascular caliber, other investigators tried to distinguish different GC phenotypes according to the microvascular patterns. Nakayoshi and colleagues[36] classified the microvascular patterns of GC into 3 groups by using magnification combined with NBI: group A, fine network; group B, corkscrew; and group C, unclassified. Depressed differentiated GC was more likely to exhibit a fine network pattern, whereas undifferentiated GC was more likely to exhibit a corkscrew pattern. However, there were still 41% of the cases that could not be classified. Although magnification endoscopy combined with NBI seems to be superior to conventional endoscopy, a systematic review suggested that the consequences of its application are limited.[44]

Other virtual chromoendoscopy technologies, such as FICE system (Fujinon, Wayne, USA) and i-Scan system (Pentax, Tokyo, Japan), were also applied in the diagnosis of EGC but their efficacy is under study. Available data indicate that virtual chromoendoscopy improves the visualization of EGC.[41]

In summary, chromoendoscopy with conventional endoscopy and virtual chromoendoscopy are helpful in the detection of EGC. Magnification endoscopy combined with NBI not only increases the detection rate of EGC but also distinguishes different histologic phenotypes according to microvascular architecture. However, analysis of microvessels by NBI could not be performed without first obtaining a clear image of the blood vessels in some patients. Gastric pit pattern assessment by using enhanced magnification endoscopy seems to be both sensitive and specific but has poor positive predictive value. Histology remains the gold standard for diagnosis of GC.

Endomicroscopy of GC

Identification of GC by Endomicroscopy

At present, the in vivo CLE features of GC are based on fluorescein sodium staining. In vivo characterization of GC mainly consists of 3 aspects: cell, tissue structure, and microvessel.[32] Although all the studies on in vivo diagnosis of GC by using CLE revealed excellent sensitivity from 81.8% to 92.6% and specificity from 99.4% to 100%,[10,12,13] the diagnostic systems applied in these studies are not unified. The descriptions of in vivo CLE imaging of GC by Kakeji and colleagues[12] mainly involve irregular variable-sized cancer cells and irregular bizarre-looking vessels. Kitabatake and colleagues[13] paid much attention to the deformation of tissue structure, such as disorganized configuration of glands and variable shapes of ductal structures. According to Zhang and colleagues'[10] classification of gastric pit patterns by CLE, type G having atypical cells or glands without normal pits. For the diagnosis of GC, type G had a sensitivity of 90%, a specificity of 99.4%, an accuracy of 97.1%, a positive predictive value of 85.7%, and a negative predictive value of 97.6%. Liu and colleagues'[14] report focused on the altered microvessels. Unlike the regular honeycomblike microvessels in the gastric body and the coil-shaped microvessels in the antrum, the microvessels in GC are irregular in shape, number, and distribution. The differences among the diagnostic systems may be because of differences in observers' preferences and sample selection. Systematic integrated diagnostic criteria should be recommended, which is summarized in **Table 1**.

Although alterations of nuclei are the hallmarks of neoplasia or dysplasia, in vivo assessment of nuclei in gastric mucosa is not practical so far. The nuclei staining agent acriflavine, unlike fluorescein sodium routinely used in fundus angiography, is at present limited to the study of ex vivo CLE imaging of gastric mucosa. In the study of the ex vivo gastric tissue by Kakeji and colleagues,[12] the mean nuclear area of cancer cells was found to be significantly larger than that of normal cells. Other parameters, such as cytologic (variably sized and enlarged nuclei, rounded nuclei, loss of polarity, prominent nucleoli) and architectural changes (complex budding or branching of glands, back-to-back glands), could also be evaluated in the ex vivo CLE observation. The in vivo nuclei assessment by using CLE might be achieved in the future by the application of well-proven nontoxic nuclei staining agents.

Classification of GC by Endomicroscopy

Endoscopic classification of GC is important for management and prognosis prediction. The 2 types of GC display distinct features in CLE images, which allows for real-time phenotypic diagnosis. In Zhang and colleagues'[10] classification of gastric pit patterns by using CLE, type G was divided into 2 subtypes, G1 and G2. Subtype G1 represents undifferentiated adenocarcinoma with atypical cells, which have no gland organization. Subtype G2 represents differentiated adenocarcinoma with atypical glands. This finding was similar to the descriptions by Kitabatake and colleagues,[13] in which differentiated GC was shown as having disorganized configuration of glands, whereas undifferentiated GC was shown as having diffusely proliferating atypical cells without ductal structures. Interpretation of the CLE images by 2 pathologists revealed accurate prediction of the histology, with excellent interobserver agreement. Both pathologists also accurately interpreted the CLE images with regard to the grade of differentiation.[13]

Besides tissue structure analysis, microvessels in differentiated and undifferentiated adenocarcinoma also display distinct features. The increased number of small vessels were tortuous, dilated, irregular in shape, and were of various diameters. In contrast, undifferentiated intramucosal cancers indicated that hypovascularity and irregular short branched or twiglike tumor vessels did not interconnect.[14] CLE images of different phenotypes of GC and the corresponding histology of the phenotypes are shown in **Fig. 2**.

According to the statements of Morson and Dawson,[23] to be of maximum benefit, a histologic classification of tumors should fulfill 3 criteria:

1. It should be easy to apply and reproducible.
2. It should help in the assessment of the prognosis.
3. It should relate to the histogenesis and if possible the cause of the tumor types.

Table 1 Diagnosis of GC by using CLE			
	Tissue Structure	**Cells**	**Microvessels**
Normal	Surface patterns of gastric types	Regular and orderly columnar cells	Normal caliber and regular
GC	Disorganized or destroyed architecture	Irregular and disordered cells	Increased caliber and irregular

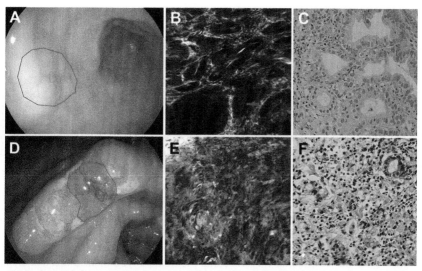

Fig. 2. Endoscopic images, CLE images, and corresponding histology of GC. (*A*) Endoscopic image shows a slightly elevated lesion with depressed center in the gastric antrum. (*B*) CLE image shows replacement of normal pits by irregular glands with distorted duct. The dilated and distorted microvascular network is visible (*arrow*). (*C*) The cross-sectional hematoxylin-eosin–stained histology shows irregular glands covered by atypical cells confirming a differentiated adenocarcinoma (HE, ×400). (*D*) Endoscopic image of a depressed lesion on the gastric angle shows destructed pit patterns different from the surrounding mucosa. (*E*) CLE image shows absence of glands and presence of atypical cells. Microvascular network is absent with only a short branch of microvessel (*arrow*). (*F*) The cross-sectional hematoxylin-eosin–stained histology shows diffusely atypical cells confirming a signet ring cell carcinoma (HE, ×400).

However, none of the current histologic classifications satisfy all these criteria.[23] Therefore, further studies of the endomicroscopic classification of GC are needed.

ENDOCYTOSCOPY

Although endocytoscopy is another important endomicroscopic technology, its application was mostly studied on the diagnosis of esophageal and colorectal diseases. A case report of signet ring cell carcinoma indicated that endocytoscopic features correlate well with those of histology. However, the images of the case were acquired from ex vivo study.[45] The in vivo diagnostic yield needs to be further confirmed.

LIMITATIONS

Despite its promising potential in in vivo diagnosis of GIM and GC, CLE as an endoscopic technique at present has some disadvantages: (1) the lack of red flag function makes CLE not superior to conventional endoscopy in detecting small and inapparent lesions and (2) the too small vision of CLE (475 × 475 μm) makes it difficult to give a complete evaluation of large areas. These disadvantages may be overcome by combined virtual chromoendoscopy or magnification endoscopy capabilities into next generations of CLE.

SUMMARY

In conclusion, the in vivo diagnosis of GIM and GC by using CLE is promising. CLE features of GIM include goblet cells, columnar absorptive cells and brush border, and villiform foveolar epithelium. CLE images of GIM could be further divided into complete and incomplete types based on the shape of goblet cells, the presence of absorptive cells or brush border, and the architecture of vessels and crypts. CLE features of GC include atypical cells, disorganized gastric pits and glands, and irregular bizarre-looking microvessels. CLE images of GC could be further divided into differentiated and undifferentiated adenocarcinomas. The former has distorted gland organization with hypervascularity, whereas the latter has no gland organization with hypovascularity.

REFERENCES

1. Correa P. A human model of gastric carcinogenesis. Cancer Res 1988;48(13): 3554–60.
2. Rokkas T, Filipe MI, Sladen GE. Detection of an increased incidence of early gastric cancer in patients with intestinal metaplasia type III who are closely followed up. Gut 1991;32(10):1110–3.
3. Dinis-Ribeiro M, da Costa-Pereira A, Lopes C, et al. Magnification chromoendoscopy for the diagnosis of gastric intestinal metaplasia and dysplasia. Gastrointest Endosc 2003;57(4):498–504.
4. Yang JM, Chen L, Fan YL, et al. Endoscopic patterns of gastric mucosa and its clinicopathological significance. World J Gastroenterol 2003;9(11):2552–6.
5. Meining A, Rosch T, Kiesslich R, et al. Inter- and intra-observer variability of magnification chromoendoscopy for detecting specialized intestinal metaplasia at the gastroesophageal junction. Endoscopy 2004;36(2):160–4.
6. Tanaka K, Toyoda H, Kadowaki S, et al. Surface pattern classification by enhanced-magnification endoscopy for identifying early gastric cancers. Gastrointest Endosc 2008;67(3):430–7.
7. Kiesslich R, Burg J, Vieth M, et al. Confocal laser endoscopy for diagnosing intraepithelial neoplasias and colorectal cancer in vivo. Gastroenterology 2004; 127(3):706–13.
8. Kiesslich R, Goetz M, Vieth M, et al. Confocal laser endomicroscopy. Gastrointest Endosc Clin N Am 2005;15(4):715–31.
9. Goetz M, Hoffman A, Galle PR, et al. Confocal laser endoscopy: new approach to the early diagnosis of tumors of the esophagus and stomach. Future Oncol 2006; 2(4):469–76.
10. Zhang JN, Li YQ, Zhao YA, et al. Classification of gastric pit patterns by confocal endomicroscopy. Gastrointest Endosc 2008;67(6):843–53.
11. Guo YT, Li YQ, Yu T, et al. Diagnosis of gastric intestinal metaplasia with confocal laser endomicroscopy in vivo: a prospective study. Endoscopy 2008;40(7): 547–53.
12. Kakeji Y, Yamaguchi S, Yoshida D, et al. Development and assessment of morphologic criteria for diagnosing gastric cancer using confocal endomicroscopy: an ex vivo and in vivo study. Endoscopy 2006;38(9):886–90.
13. Kitabatake S, Niwa Y, Miyahara R, et al. Confocal endomicroscopy for the diagnosis of gastric cancer in vivo. Endoscopy 2006;38(11):1110–4.
14. Liu H, Li YQ, Yu T, et al. Confocal endomicroscopy for in vivo detection of microvascular architecture in normal and malignant lesions of upper gastrointestinal tract. J Gastroenterol Hepatol 2008;23(1):56–61.

15. Kiesslich R, Canto MI. Confocal laser endomicroscopy. Gastrointest Endosc Clin N Am 2009;19(2):261–72.
16. Odagi I, Kato T, Imazu H, et al. Examination of normal intestine using confocal endomicroscopy. J Gastroenterol Hepatol 2007;22(5):658–62.
17. Kiesslich R, Gotz M, Neurath MF, et al. [Endomicroscopy–technology with future]. Internist (Berl) 2006;47(1):8–17 [in German].
18. Sanduleanu S, Driessen A, Gomez-Garcia E, et al. In vivo diagnosis and classification of colorectal neoplasia by chromoendoscopy-guided confocal laser endomicroscopy. Clin Gastroenterol Hepatol 2010;8(4):371–8.
19. Goetz M, Toermer T, Vieth M, et al. Simultaneous confocal laser endomicroscopy and chromoendoscopy with topical cresyl violet. Gastrointest Endosc 2009; 70(5):959–68.
20. Toyoda H, Rubio C, Befrits R, et al. Detection of intestinal metaplasia in distal esophagus and esophagogastric junction by enhanced-magnification endoscopy. Gastrointest Endosc 2004;59(1):15–21.
21. Gheorghe C. Narrow-band imaging endoscopy for diagnosis of malignant and premalignant gastrointestinal lesions. J Gastrointestin Liver Dis 2006;15(1):77–82.
22. Evans JA, Bouma BE, Bressner J, et al. Identifying intestinal metaplasia at the squamocolumnar junction by using optical coherence tomography. Gastrointest Endosc 2007;65(1):50–6.
23. Morson BC, Dawson IMP. Morson and Dawson's gastrointestinal pathology. 3rd editon. Oxford (Oxfordshire): Blackwell Scientific; 1990.
24. Teglbjaerg PS, Nielsen HO. "Small intestinal type" and "colonic type" intestinal metaplasia of the human stomach, and their relationship to the histogenetic types of gastric adenocarcinoma. Acta Pathol Microbiol Scand A Am 1978;86(5):351–5.
25. Sipponen P, Seppala K, Varis K, et al. Intestinal metaplasia with colonic-type sulphomucins in the gastric mucosa; its association with gastric carcinoma. Acta Pathol Microbiol Scand A 1980;88(4):217–24.
26. Ramesar KC, Sanders DS, Hopwood D. Limited value of type III intestinal metaplasia in predicting risk of gastric carcinoma. J Clin Pathol 1987;40(11):1287–90.
27. Guelrud M, Herrera I, Essenfeld H, et al. Intestinal metaplasia of the gastric cardia: a prospective study with enhanced magnification endoscopy. Am J Gastroenterol 2002;97(3):584–9.
28. Uedo N, Ishihara R, Iishi H, et al. A new method of diagnosing gastric intestinal metaplasia: narrow-band imaging with magnifying endoscopy. Endoscopy 2006; 38(8):819–24.
29. Dinis-Ribeiro M, da Costa-Pereira A, Lopes C, et al. Feasibility and cost-effectiveness of using magnification chromoendoscopy and pepsinogen serum levels for the follow-up of patients with atrophic chronic gastritis and intestinal metaplasia. J Gastroenterol Hepatol 2007;22(10):1594–604.
30. Areia M, Amaro P, Dinis-Ribeiro M, et al. External validation of a classification for methylene blue magnification chromoendoscopy in premalignant gastric lesions. Gastrointest Endosc 2008;67(7):1011–8.
31. Olliver JR, Wild CP, Sahay P, et al. Chromoendoscopy with methylene blue and associated DNA damage in Barrett's oesophagus. Lancet 2003;362(9381):373–4.
32. Kiesslich R, Galle PR, Neurath M. Atlas of endomicroscopy. SpringerLink (online service). Berlin: Springer Medizin Verlag Heidelberg; 2008. Available at: http://dx. doi.org/10.1007/978-3-540-35115-3. Accessed August 17, 2010.
33. Bao H, Boussioutas A, Reynolds J, et al. Imaging of goblet cells as a marker for intestinal metaplasia of the stomach by one-photon and two-photon fluorescence endomicroscopy. J Biomed Opt 2009;14(6):064031.

34. Ralf K, Maximilian S, Lee Guan L, et al. T1620: endomicroscopy is able to identify superficial but not deep intestinal metaplasia of the gastric mucosa. Gastrointest Endosc 2010;71(5):AB324.

35. Roukos D, Lorenz M, Hottenrott C. [Prognostic significance of the Lauren classification of patients with stomach carcinoma. A statistical analysis of long-term results following gastrectomy]. Schweiz Med Wochenschr 1989;119(21):755–9 [in German].

36. Nakayoshi T, Tajiri H, Matsuda K, et al. Magnifying endoscopy combined with narrow band imaging system for early gastric cancer: correlation of vascular pattern with histopathology (including video). Endoscopy 2004;36(12):1080–4.

37. Ohashi A, Niwa Y, Ohmiya N, et al. Quantitative analysis of the microvascular architecture observed on magnification endoscopy in cancerous and benign gastric lesions. Endoscopy 2005;37(12):1215–9.

38. Dinis-Ribeiro M. Chromoendoscopy for early diagnosis of gastric cancer. Eur J Gastroenterol Hepatol 2006;18(8):831–8.

39. Tanaka K, Toyoda H, Kadowaki S, et al. Features of early gastric cancer and gastric adenoma by enhanced-magnification endoscopy. J Gastroenterol 2006; 41(4):332–8.

40. Yao K, Iwashita A, Tanabe H, et al. White opaque substance within superficial elevated gastric neoplasia as visualized by magnification endoscopy with narrow-band imaging: a new optical sign for differentiating between adenoma and carcinoma. Gastrointest Endosc 2008;68(3):574–80.

41. Mouri R, Yoshida S, Tanaka S, et al. Evaluation and validation of computed virtual chromoendoscopy in early gastric cancer. Gastrointest Endosc 2009;69(6):1052–8.

42. Ezoe Y, Muto M, Horimatsu T, et al. Magnifying narrow-band imaging versus magnifying white-light imaging for the differential diagnosis of gastric small depressive lesions: a prospective study. Gastrointest Endosc 2010;71(3):477–84.

43. Tahara T, Shibata T, Nakamura M, et al. The mucosal pattern in the non-neoplastic gastric mucosa by using magnifying narrow-band imaging endoscopy significantly correlates with gastric cancer risk. Gastrointest Endosc 2010;71(2):429–30.

44. Curvers WL, van den Broek FJ, Reitsma JB, et al. Systematic review of narrow-band imaging for the detection and differentiation of abnormalities in the esophagus and stomach (with video). Gastrointest Endosc 2009;69(2):307–17.

45. Fasoli A, Pugliese V, Furnari M, et al. Signet ring cell carcinoma of the stomach: correlation between endocytoscopy and histology. Endoscopy 2009;41(Suppl 2): E65–6.

How to Approach the Small Bowel with Flexible Enteroscopy

Andrea May, MD, PhD

KEYWORDS

- Push enteroscopy • Double balloon enteroscopy
- Single balloon enteroscopy • Balloon-assisted enteroscopy
- Spiral enteroscopy • Small bowel endoscopy

Flexible enteroscopy is a more invasive procedure in comparison with the purely diagnostic capsule endoscopy. However, the main advantages of flexible enteroscopy in comparison with other imaging procedures (eg, capsule endoscopy and magnetic resonance Sellink) are that it allows histologic sampling and endoscopic therapy. Nowadays, several techniques are available for the approach of the small bowel, including push enteroscopy (PE), balloon-assisted enteroscopy (BAE) using 2 balloons (double-balloon enteroscopy [DBE]) or 1 balloon (single-balloon enteroscopy [SBE]), balloon-guided enteroscopy (BGE), and spiral enteroscopy (SE). PE became established in the 1980s but is associated with only a limited depth of penetration into the small bowel. This limitation was overcome through the development of BAE using the DBE or SBE technique.[1–4] In optimal cases, the entire small bowel, or at least considerable proportions of it, can be visualized using balloon enteroscopy (usually by combining the oral and anal examinations). This system has become established throughout the world for diagnostic and therapeutic small bowel examinations and is now being used universally in clinical routine work. In addition to the classic indication for small bowel endoscopy, the DBE or SBE technique has a variety of other potential uses as well, for example, in difficult ileocolonoscopies, for access to the pancreatic and biliary tract in patients with a surgically modified gastrointestinal tract, and for access to the stomach in patients who have undergone bariatric surgery. SE is another promising recently introduced enteroscopic system that is equipped with a raised helix at the tip of the overtube.[5] In contrast to the BAE techniques, which follow the push-and-pull principle, this new enteroscopic technique pleats the small bowel by rotating.

Department of Internal Medicine II, HSK Wiesbaden, Ludwig-Erhard-Strasse 100, 65199 Wiesbaden, Germany
E-mail address: andrea.may@hsk-wiesbaden.de

Gastroenterol Clin N Am 39 (2010) 797–806
doi:10.1016/j.gtc.2010.08.024
0889-8553/10/$ – see front matter © 2010 Elsevier Inc. All rights reserved.

FLEXIBLE ENTEROSCOPIC TECHNIQUES
PE

Push video enteroscopes are 200- to 250-cm long devices (dependent on type and manufacturer) and might be used with a stiff overtube (85–120 cm) to prevent looping of the enteroscope in the stomach. Although initial studies showed an increase in the depth of insertion with the use of an overtube,[6,7] later studies with graded-stiffness enteroscopes have questioned the additional value of the overtube.[8,9] The following are the main advantages of PE: it is easy and quick to perform, it is not a staff-consuming procedure, the overtube is reusable, and there is no need to set up a special system (eg, a pump control system). All these facts avoid extra costs and, therefore, PE is a cost-saving technique for the investigation of the proximal small bowel.[1] PE for the lower digestive tract is not commonly performed because insertion depth of colonoscopy with ileoscopy seems equivalent to lower PE.[10]

BAE

DBE

The DBE system (Fujinon, Inc, Saitama, Japan) consists of a high-resolution video endoscope with a working length of 200 cm and a flexible overtube made of polyure-thane. Latex balloons are attached both at the tip of the enteroscope and also on the overtube and they can be inflated with air or deflated using a pressure-controlled pump. At present, 3 different types of devices are available with the DBE system. First type is the EN450-P5 model with a working channel of 2.2 mm and an outer diameter of 8.5 mm. Second is the EN450-T5 model with a working channel of 2.8 mm and an outer diameter of 9.4 mm. The corresponding overtubes have diameters of 12.2 and 13.2 mm with an overall length of 145 cm. Third is the EC450-BI5 model with a length of 152 cm, an outer diameter of 9.4 mm, a working channel of 2.8 mm, and a corre-sponding overtube with a diameter of 13.2 mm and a length of 110 cm. This device is mainly used for difficult ileocolonoscopy, endoscopic retrograde cholangiopancrea-tography in surgically altered anatomy, or proximal small bowel endoscopy. The main advantage is that there is no need for specially designed accessories, and all standard equipment can be used.

The principle of the DBE technique is based on alternating pushing and pulling maneuvers and alternating inflation and deflation of the balloons, allowing the small bowel to be threaded step-by-step onto the overtube (**Fig. 1**).[4,5] Depending on the

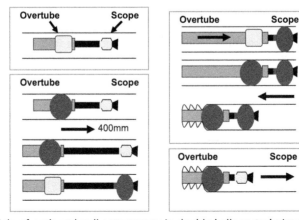

Fig. 1. Principle of push-and-pull enteroscopy in double-balloon technique.

intention, the pleated small bowel can slip down very fast or slowly from the overtube during withdrawal, using the alternating inflation and deflation of the overtube balloon while pulling back the scope. To optimize the visualization, the balloon at the endoscope tip is used in addition to air insufflation, if necessary. The endoscope balloon can then be partly inflated to a balloon setting pressure of 4 to 5 kPa, helping to pull apart the pleated folds.

SBE

The SBE system was introduced as a simplification of the DBE device. The enteroscope (XSIF Q160Y or SIF-Q180 [Olympus Optical Co, Tokyo, Japan]) is also a high-resolution video endoscope, with a working length of 200 cm. The enteroscope is equipped with a working channel of 2.8 mm diameter and its outer diameter is 9.2 mm. The overtube has an overall length of 140 cm and consists of silicone as well as the balloon at its distal end. In contrast to the DBE system, the balloon is not attached to the tip of the enteroscope, and stable positioning in the small bowel, for example, during advance of the overtube, is achieved by angling the tip of the endoscope or by the so-called power suction.[4,11] Insufflation of the overtube balloon is performed using a pressure-controlled pump. The small bowel is threaded step-by-step onto the overtube and by alternating pushing and pulling maneuvers.

In principle, the DBE system can also be used as an SBE technique by dispensing with the balloon attached to the enteroscope tip (**Fig. 2**).[12,13]

BGE

The BGE system (NaviAid BGE, Smart Medical Systems Ltd, Israel) enables enteroscopy with standard endoscopes and endoscopic equipment. The BGE device comprises a 2-balloon add-on disposable element and an air supply unit to control the inflation and deflation of the balloons.[14] The BGE also follows the push-and-pull principle, but in contrast to DBE and SBE, the guidance during advancement into the small bowel is taken by the balloon, not by the endoscope.

SE

For SE, a special overtube called Discovery Small Bowel (Spirus Medical Inc, Stoughton, MA, USA) has to be used. This overtube consists of polyvinyl chloride and has a length of 118 cm, an outer diameter of 16 mm, and an internal diameter of 9.8 mm. Therefore, both the slim enteroscopes manufactured by Fujinon and Olympus (without overtube or balloon) can be used for SE. The tip of the overtube has a raised hollow spiral that is 5.5 mm high over a length of 21 cm (**Fig. 3**). In addition, the overtube has 2 handles for manual rotation, a locking device at the proximal part, and an injection port for lubrication. A special jelly has to be used for lubrication.

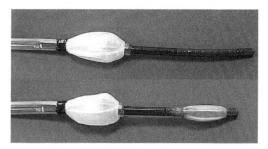

Fig. 2. Push-and-pull enteroscopy using single and double-balloon technique.

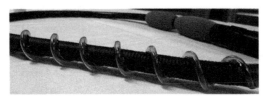

Fig. 3. Spiral overtube with raised helix at the tip.

By clockwise rotation of the overtube, the small bowel is pleated onto the overtube, and for withdrawal, counterclockwise rotation is performed.

EXAMINATION PROCEDURE
Preparation

For all deep small bowel endoscopic techniques, the patients generally only needed to fast before the oral examination (approximately 10–12 hours for food and 2–4 hours for clear liquids). Laxative measures before oral examinations should only be performed in patients with signs of intestinal obstruction or with diabetic neuropathy with delayed transit. For the anal examination, patients should undergo bowel preparation in the same way as for colonoscopy, including splitting, which means taking half of the bowel cleansing solution on the day before enteroscopy and half on the day of the enteroscopy. In patients with constipation or other motility disorders, intensification of the laxative preparation is recommended.

Sedation

Depending on the condition of the patient (eg, age, comorbidities), most examinations can be performed with the patients under conscious sedation in the same way as in colonoscopy and upper gastrointestinal tract endoscopy. For difficult and long investigations or patients who are difficult to handle with conscious sedation, propofol can be used as an alternative. For SE, propofol-based sedation is recommended. General anesthesia with intubation is not customary in Germany and is restricted to individual cases, for example, in children. But in other countries, general anesthesia with intubation is used more often. There is a wide range of sedation options and their selection is related to local conditions and policies.

CO_2 Insufflation

A previous prospective 2-center study demonstrated substantial advantages with regard to patient comfort and insertion depth with the use of CO_2 insufflation instead of air insufflation in DBE.[15] Despite these positive data, however, the use of CO_2 has not yet become generally established.

Fluoroscopy

Depending on the experience of the endoscopist and the patient's anatomic conditions, radiological fluoroscopy can be used optionally in flexible enteroscopy. Particularly, in the case of adhesions after abdominal surgeries, fluoroscopy is very useful.[16,17] When stenoses are expected, for example, in patients with Crohn disease, radiology is certainly useful because the radiographic contrast image allows good assessment of the complexity of impassable stenoses.

Therapeutic Interventions

Therapeutic interventions should be generally performed during withdrawal of the instrument to avoid perforation caused by stretching of the small bowel wall during push-and-pull maneuvers or rotation. Endoscopic treatment of angiodysplasias or vascular malformations can be performed during endoscope advancement only if capsule endoscopy had previously shown a solitary or only very few small lesions (<5) to prevent the lesions from being missed between the threaded folds during withdrawal. During withdrawal of the endoscope and therapeutic interventions, spasmolytics improve visualization of the small bowel mucosa by reducing peristalsis of the small bowel. Because of the length of the enteroscopes and loop formation within the small bowel, insertion of accessories through the working channel might be troublesome. In these cases, straightening of the enteroscope position or the flexed enteroscope tip as well as enlargement of small cramped loops under fluoroscopic control is helpful. In addition, lubrication of the working channel with, for example, silicon oil, is recommended to facilitate insertion of devices through the working channel.[18]

In Germany, therapeutic examinations are performed on an inpatient basis, but there might be different ways of management in different countries. Patients should be inquired about symptoms approximately 4 hours after the end of the examination as well as the next day. The method to allow patients only to drink water or tea until the next morning after therapy proved to be worthwhile in the author's experience.

Measurement of Insertion

PE cannot evaluate the nonoperated small bowel in its entire length, and generally, the reported insertion depths from the oral route are given as postpyloric distance. If an overtube is used, the overtube is held in a stable position during advancement of the enteroscope to avoid looping in the stomach. The enteroscope is inserted as far as possible into the small bowel. After straightening, the scope is pulled back until the pylorus is reached again. The distance in centimeters between the pylorus and the deepest point after straightening of the scope is measured as the insertion depth.[1] In the same way, the distance past the ligament of Treitz can be measured.

All BAE techniques follow the push-and-pull principle. The insertion depth of the endoscope into the small bowel is estimated by recording the net advancement of the endoscope for each push-and-pull maneuver on a standardized documentation sheet. In other words, the endoscopist has to estimate the effective insertion length of the enteroscope by the endoscopic checking of the instrument's advancement and the length of small bowel released during insertion of the overtube and pulling back of the enteroscope and overtube. At the end of the examination, all the individual lengths advanced are added up. This technique requires some experience but it has been evaluated using an animal model.[19] For SBE with an inverted tip technique, this measurement might not be feasible because during the pull maneuver, the angulated tip of the endoscope obstructs the view and makes it more difficult to estimate the length of each step.

In contrast to the push-and-pull enteroscopic techniques, which measure the insertion depths step-by-step on intubation, the insertion depth during SE is estimated on withdrawal.[5] In other words, the endoscopist has to estimate how much small bowel is released from the overtube on the way back, which might be done in a reliable way by experienced and model-trained enteroscopists.[5] But generally it is only a very rough estimation, which is even more susceptible to bias than the step-by-step measurement of DBE. This estimation is problematic for trials comparing insertion depths of the different enteroscopic techniques. Therefore, the only objective parameter is the rate of complete enteroscopy.

COMPLICATIONS
PE

Complications such as mucosal stripping, perforation, and pancreatitis that have been reported with PE were caused by the overtube and mainly observed in the duodenum.[20–22] To minimize the risk of complications, PE can be performed without the overtube or the overtube can be positioned in front of the pylorus, without passing the pylorus. In a prospective comparison of PE and DBE, the overtube was not pushed into the duodenum and this is probably the reason why there was no complication in the small bowel and no cases of pancreatitis.[1]

BAE (DBE and SBE)

Most of the data exist for DBE, including the German double-balloon registry with just less than 4000 DBE procedures, a US data collection of just less than 2500 DBE procedures, and a European data collection of just less than 2400 DBE procedures.[23–25] From the published data, relevant overall complications in DBE can be expected in approximately 1% of cases. The most severe complication in diagnostic DBE is certainly pancreatitis, with a risk of approximately 0.2% to 0.3% in oral DBE. As in conventional endoscopy, the risk of severe complications is higher in therapeutic enteroscopy, which is at around 3% to 4%.[18,23,25] With regard to the mortality rate associated with DBE, the only data available are from the German double-balloon registry.[23] The mortality rate here is 0.05% (death after pancreatitis and complicated postoperative course after perforation during polypectomy for a small bowel polyp).

At present, fewer data are available with regard to the expected complication rates in diagnostic and therapeutic SBE. The risk of deep mucosal tears or the risk of perforation (up to 2.3%) as a severe complication of a diagnostic examination[4,26–28] might be higher if the endoscope tip is flexed during the advancement of the overtube, especially in the case of adhesions caused by prior abdominal surgery or anastomotic strictures. The technique of power suction[11] might help to reduce the injuries caused by the inverted endoscope tip technique, because power suction was the preferred technique in a prospective comparison of DBE and SBE, without any severe complications for both DBE and SBE.[29] Altogether, the number of patients in the studies on SBE is too small to make a meaningful comparison with the huge number of data of DBE. However, it can be assumed that the complication rates of diagnostic SBE are similar to those of diagnostic DBE because of the fact that both the techniques follow the same push-and-pull principle. The same can be expected for therapeutic interventions.[30]

SE

At present, limited data are available with regard to the expected complication rates in diagnostic and therapeutic SE. In contrast to the diagnostic DBE with acute pancreatitis as the leading severe complication, perforation seems to be the leading severe complication in diagnostic SE, with 0.34% (6/1750) in a retrospective analysis of 1750 patients and up to 3.5% (1/28) in elderly patients.[31,32] Especially, the geriatric patients (>65 years) might be a group with increased risk for severe complications, altogether 6.5% with 1 fatal outcome.[32] But the limited data are contradictory because in another study of patients with a mean age of 65 years and comorbidities, no perforations occurred.[33] For a reliable assessment, further prospective studies with SE are needed.

COMPARISON OF THE DIFFERENT ENTEROSCOPIC TECHNIQUES

A prospective study in patients with suspected midgastrointestinal bleeding showed that DBE was superior to PE for endoscopic examination of the small bowel, both with regard to the length of the small bowel visualized and the diagnostic yield.[1] PE is a cost-saving, easy, and fast procedure for the examination of the proximal jejunum, but for deeper small endoscopy, the other techniques are required.

There are only preliminary data published on BGE, and no comparing studies exist. BGE advancement was deeper than in the published results for PE, although not equaling that in DBE.[14] But the balloon guidance, instead of endoscope guidance, makes insertion difficult, especially in the deeper parts of the small bowel and in case of sharp bends or adhesions caused by prior abdominal surgery. Therefore, it could be expected that BGE is less effective regarding the insertion depth when compared with BAE or SE.

Comparing DBE and SBE based on the published literature, the diagnostic yield of DBE, at around 60% to 80%, seems to be higher than that of SBE, at around 40% to 60%. Most publications on DBE have reported a high rate of endoscopic interventions, between 35% and 65%, whereas the rate of endoscopic interventions during SBE was only from 5% to 24%.[4,26,27,34–41] One prospective multicenter trial comparing the DBE and SBE techniques using the Fujinon device showed that the DBE technique was clearly superior to the SBE technique.[29] The rate of complete enteroscopy was 3 times higher in the DBE group than the SBE group (66% vs 22%), with a higher overall diagnostic and therapeutic yield in the DBE group of 72% versus 48% in the SBE group.

No prospective randomized studies comparing SE with DBE or SBE have been published so far. The low diagnostic yield of relevant pathologies in the small bowel of 9% to 24% associated with a low rate of endoscopic therapy of up to 13% in the first 2 SE studies can be explained by the feasibility of these studies.[5,42] With better patient selection, the diagnostic yield is increasing (59%–65%), as well as therapeutic interventions.[33,43] The main advantage of SE is that the average investigation time can be decreased to around 40 to 45 minutes,[33,43,44] which is definitely shorter than the mean investigation times reported for BAE with around 50 to 90 minutes.[1,4,16,28–30,35–37,41,45] In addition, the stability of endoscopic view during the controlled withdrawal by counterclockwise rotation of the stiff overtube is satisfying and facilitates endoscopic interventions (author's experience). The main disadvantage of SE is the very low rate of complete enteroscopy, which is increasingly important. Actually, only 2 cases are reported: one with the oral route alone and one with combined oral and anal approaches.[43,46] Even if complete enteroscopy is possible within 1 oral session, a combination of the oral and anal examination is necessary in most patients,

Table 1 Comparison of BAE (DBE and SBE) and SE			
	DBE	SBE	SE
Diagnostic yield	~60%–80%	~40%–60%	~10%–65%
Therapeutic interventions	~35%–65%	~5%–25%	<5%–50%
Complete enteroscopy	~35%–80%	~10%–25%	<1% (?)
Complications			
Diagnostic enteroscopy	~1%	0%–2%	0%–6.5%
Therapeutic enteroscopy	~3%–4%	–5%	?

Rounded numbers.

in whom a total enteroscopy is attempted. But the effectiveness of anal SE is still uncertain because the passage through the colon is generally easy, but insertion of the enteroscope and the overtube through the ileocecal valve is difficult and therefore results in limited insertion depths into the distal small bowel. A maximum anal insertion depth of 130 cm is reported in SE (author's experience),[46] which is much lower than the maximum insertion depths of 320 to 370 cm reported for DBE.[35–37,39] Furthermore, it seems that in case of adhesions, SE is even more difficult to perform than BAE (author's experience).[44] Comparative data of the different enteroscopy techniques are listed in **Table 1**.

SUMMARY

PE is a cost-saving, easy, and fast procedure for examination of the proximal jejunum, but for deeper small endoscopy, the other flexible enteroscopic techniques are required. Actually, 4 different systems are available: BAE with DBE and SBE, BGE, and SE.

BGE does not play a considerable role in deep small bowel endoscopy. DBE is the oldest flexible enteroscopic technique and has become established throughout the world for diagnostic and therapeutic examinations of the small bowel. DBE is still regarded as the gold standard nonsurgical procedure for deep small bowel endoscopy, because it provides the highest rates of complete enteroscopy, which becomes increasingly useful. The recently introduced SE technique represents a promising method but still needs technical improvement. Larger prospective studies on SE and prospective studies comparing the 3 systems (DBE, SBE, SE) are awaited before conclusive assessments can be made. In future, the physicians probably have to decide from case to case, depending on the intention of the examination and the patient's conditions, on which method to choose, because every enteroscopic technique has advantages and disadvantages. It is more important to have endoscopic centers with experience in different enteroscopic techniques.

REFERENCES

1. May A, Nachbar L, Schneider M, et al. Prospective comparison of push enteroscopy and push-and-pull enteroscopy in patients with suspected small-bowel bleeding. Am J Gastroenterol 2006;101:2016–24.
2. Yamamoto H, Sekine Y, Sato Y, et al. Total enteroscopy with a nonsurgical steerable double-balloon method. Gastrointest Endosc 2001;53:216–20.
3. May A, Nachbar L, Wardak A, et al. Double-balloon enteroscopy: preliminary experience in patients with obscure gastrointestinal bleeding or chronic abdominal pain. Endoscopy 2003;35:985–91.
4. Tsujikawa T, Saitoh Y, Andoh A, et al. Novel single-balloon enteroscopy for diagnosis and treatment of the small intestine: preliminary experiences. Endoscopy 2008;40:11–5.
5. Akerman P, Agrawal D, Cantero D, et al. Spiral enteroscopy with the new DSB overtube: a novel technique for deep peroral small bowel intubation. Endoscopy 2008;40:974–8.
6. Taylor AC, Chen RY, Desmond PV. Use of an overtube for enteroscopy – does it increase depth of insertion? A prospective study of enteroscopy with and without an overtube. Endoscopy 2001;33:227–30.
7. Iida M, Yamamoto T, Yao T, et al. Jejunal endoscopy using a long duodenofiberscope. Gastrointest Endosc 1986;32:233–6.
8. Keizman D, Brill S, Umansky M, et al. Diagnostic yield of routine push enteroscopy with a graded-stiffness enteroscope without overtube. Gastrointest Endosc 2003;57:877–81.

9. Lin S, Branch MS, Shetzline M. The importance of indication in the diagnostic value of push enteroscopy. Endoscopy 2003;35:315–21.
10. Belaiche J, Van Kemseke C, Louis E. Use of enteroscope for colo-ileoscopy: low yield in unexplained lower gastrointestinal bleeding. Endoscopy 1999;31:298–301.
11. Kav T, Balaban Y, Bayraktar Y. The power suction maneuver in single balloon enteroscopy. Endoscopy 2008;40:961–2.
12. May A, Nachbar L, Ell C. Push-and-pull enteroscopy using a single-balloon technique for difficult colonoscopy. Endoscopy 2006;38:395–8.
13. Mönkemüller K, Fry LC, Bellutti M, et al. ERCP using single-balloon instead of double-balloon enteroscopy in patients with Roux-en-Y anastomosis. Endoscopy 2008;40:E19–20.
14. Adler SN, Bjarnason I, Metzger YC. New balloon-guided technique for deep small-intestine endoscopy using standard endoscopes. Endoscopy 2008;40:502–4.
15. Domagk D, Bretthauer M, Lenz P, et al. Carbon dioxide insufflation improves intubation depth in double-balloon enteroscopy: a randomized, controlled, double-blind trial. Endoscopy 2007;39:1064–7.
16. Mehdizadeh S, Ross A, Gerson L, et al. What is the learning curve associated with double balloon enteroscopy? Technical details and early experience in 6 US tertiary care centers. Gastrointest Endosc 2006;64:740–50.
17. Manner H, May A, Pohl J, et al. The impact of fluoroscopy on the outcome of oral double-balloon enteroscopy: results of a randomized trial in 156 patients. Endoscopy, in press.
18. May A, Nachbar L, Pohl J, et al. Endoscopic interventions in the small bowel using double-balloon enteroscopy: feasibility and limitations. Am J Gastroenterol 2007;102:527–35.
19. May A, Nachbar L, Schneider M, et al. Push-and-pull enteroscopy using the double-balloon technique: method of assessing depth of insertion and training of the enteroscopy technique using the Erlangen Endo-Trainer. Endoscopy 2005;37:66–70.
20. Landi B, Cellier C, Fayemendy L, et al. Duodenal perforation occurring during push enteroscopy [letter]. Gastrointest Endosc 1996;43:631.
21. Barkin J, Lewis B, Reiner D, et al. Diagnostic and therapeutic jejunostomy with a new, longer enteroscope. Gastrointest Endosc 1992;38:55–8.
22. Yang R, Laine L. Mucosal stripping: a complication of push enteroscopy. Gastrointest Endosc 1995;41:156–8.
23. Möschler O, May AD, Müller MK, et al. [Complications in double-balloon enteroscopy: results of the German DBE registry]. Z Gastroenterol 2008;46: 266–70 [in German].
24. Gerson LB, Batenic MA, Newsom SL, et al. Long-term outcomes after double-balloon enteroscopy for obscure gastrointestinal bleeding. Clin Gastroenterol Hepatol 2009;7:664–9.
25. Mensink P, Haringsma J, Kucharzik T, et al. Complications of double balloon enteroscopy: a multicenter survey. Endoscopy 2007;39:613–5.
26. Kawamura T, Yasuda K, Tanaka K, et al. Clinical evaluation of a newly developed single-balloon enteroscope. Gastrointest Endosc 2008;68:1112–6.
27. Tominaga K, Iida T, Nakamura Y, et al. Small-intestine perforation of endoscopically unrecognized lesions during peroral single-balloon enteroscopy. Endoscopy 2008;40(Suppl 2):E213–4.
28. Ramchandani M, Reddy DN, Gupta R, et al. Diagnostic yield and therapeutic impact of single-balloon enteroscopy: series of 106 cases. J Gastroenterol Hepatol 2009;24:1631–8.

29. May A, Färber M, Aschmoneit I, et al. Prospective multicenter trial comparing push-and-pull enteroscopy with the single- and double-balloon techniques in patients with small-bowel disorders. Am J Gastroenterol 2010;105(3):575–81.

30. Aktas H, de Ridder L, Haringsma J, et al. Complications of single-balloon enteroscopy: a prospective evaluation of 166 procedures. Endoscopy 2010;42:365–8.

31. Akerman P. Severe complications of spiral enteroscopy in the first 1750 patients. Gastrointest Endosc 2009;69:AB127–8.

32. Witkin AS, Fenkel JM, Infantolino A, et al. Spiral enteroscopy in geriatric patients: retrospective review of a single-center experience. Gastrointest Endosc 2010;71:AB.

33. Judah JR, Draganov PV, Lam Y, et al. Spiral enteroscopy is safe and effective for an elderly United States population of patients with numerous comorbidities. Clin Gastroenterol Hepatol 2010;8(7):572–6.

34. Yamamoto H, Kita H, Sunada K, et al. Clinical outcomes of double-balloon endoscopy for the diagnosis and treatment of small-intestinal diseases. Clin Gastroenterol Hepatol 2004;2:1010–6.

35. Ell C, May A, Nachbar L, et al. Push-and-pull enteroscopy in the small bowel using the double-balloon technique: results of a prospective European multicenter study. Endoscopy 2005;37:613–6.

36. May A, Nachbar L, Ell C. Double-balloon enteroscopy (push-and-pull enteroscopy) of the small bowel: feasibility and diagnostic and therapeutic yield in patients with suspected small bowel disease. Gastrointest Endosc 2005;62:62–70.

37. Heine GD, Hadithi M, Groenen MJ, et al. Double-balloon enteroscopy: indications, diagnostic yield, and complications in a series of 275 patients with suspected small-bowel disease. Endoscopy 2006;38:42–8.

38. Sun B, Rajan E, Cheng S, et al. Diagnostic yield and therapeutic impact of double-balloon enteroscopy in a large cohort of patients with obscure gastrointestinal bleeding. Am J Gastroenterol 2006;101:2011–5.

39. Zhong J, Ma T, Zhang C, et al. A retrospective study of the application on double-balloon enteroscopy in 378 patients with suspected small-bowel diseases. Endoscopy 2007;39:208–15.

40. Kuga R, Safatle-Ribeiro A, Ishida RK, et al. Small bowel endoscopy using the double-balloon technique: four-year results in a tertiary referral hospital in Brazil. Dig Dis 2008;26:318–23.

41. Frantz DJ, Dellon ES, Grimm I, et al. Single-balloon enteroscopy: results from an initial experience at a U.S. tertiary-care center. Gastrointest Endosc 2010;72(2):422–6.

42. Buscaglia JM, Dunbar KB, Okolo PI, et al. The spiral enteroscopy training initiative: results of a prospective study evaluating the Discovery SB overtube device during small bowel enteroscopy (with video). Endoscopy 2009;41:194–9.

43. Morgan D, Upchurch BR, Draganov PV, et al. Spiral enteroscopy: prospective multicenter U.S. trial in patients with small bowel disorders. Gastrointest Endosc 2009;69:AB127–8.

44. Despott EJ, Hughes S, Marden P, et al. First cases of spiral enteroscopy in the UK: let's "torque" about it! [letter to the editor]. Endoscopy 2010;42:517.

45. Despott EJ, Hughes S, Deo A, et al. Expanding the international double balloon experience: first results from the UK multi-centre DBE registry. Endoscopy 2009;41(Suppl 1):A232.

46. Lara LF, Shailender S, Sreenarasimhaiah J. Initial experience with retrograde overtube-assisted enteroscopy using a spiral tip overtube. Proc (Bayl Univ Med Cent) 2010;23:130–3.

Video Capsule Endoscopy: What Is the Future?

André Van Gossum, MD, PhD[a],*, Mostafa Ibrahim, MD[b]

KEYWORDS

- Capsule • Video capsule endoscopy • Wireless endoscopy
- Enteroscopy • Small bowel • Colon • Digestive bleeding
- Colorectal cancer screening

The introduction of wireless or video capsule endoscopy (VCE) has revolutionized imaging modalities in gastroenterology. In the last 10 years, the number of scientific publications on VCE has continuously increased, promoting a new interest for small bowel (SB) diseases.[1] Initially, VCE was used to examine the SB but was rapidly considered as a first-line procedure for several intestinal disorders. Now, the procedure is largely used in clinical practice globally.[2] Subsequently, VCE was adapted for examining the esophagus and, more recently, the colon. A new era of research and development is open. Indeed, many people believe that wireless endoscopy is still an incompletely developed technology.[3] In this article, the authors focus on the use of VCE for SB and colon diseases and describe the new and potential capabilities of VCE.

SMALL BOWEL VIDEO CAPSULE ENDOSCOPY

The VCE system comprises a capsule containing the video camera; a sensing system comprising an array of sensor pads, a data recorder, and a battery pack; and a workstation. A portable external viewer is also available for directly monitoring the images during the procedure. VCE was initially developed by Given Imaging (Yoqneam, Israel) for examining the SB (PillCam SB capsule). Subsequently, this company also developed the PillCam ESO capsule and the PillCam colon capsule for examining the esophagus and the colon, respectively. The small bowel video capsule endoscope (SBVCE) is 11 to 24–27.9 mm long, weighs approximately 3.4 to –6 g, and obtains 2 to 3 images per second. There are 5 capsule endoscopy systems available: PillCam (Given Imaging),

The authors have nothing to disclose.

[a] Department of Hepato-Gastroenterology, Erasme Hospital, Free University of Brussels, 808 Route de Lennik, Brussels 1070, Belgium

[b] Gastroenterology and Hepatology Department, Theodor Bilharz Research Institute, Cairo, Egypt

* Corresponding author.

E-mail address: Andre.vangossum@erasme.ulb.ac.be

0889-8553/10/$ – see front matter © 2010 Elsevier Inc. All rights reserved.

EndoCapsule (Olympus, Center Valley, PA, USA), MiroCam (IntroMedic, Seoul, Korea), OMOM capsule (Jinshan Science and Technology, Chongqing, China), and Sayaka (RF SYSTEM lab, Nagano, Japan); however, only PillCam and EndoCapsule are currently approved by the Food and Drug Administration (FDA) for use in the United States. Pill-Cam uses a complementary metal-oxide semiconductor (CMOS) chip, and the others use a charge-coupled device (CCD) chip for imaging (**Figs. 1–6**).

PillCam and EndoCapsule use a radiofrequency (RF)-based communication technology, whereas MiroCam is currently undergoing FDA approval trials in the United States and uses a CMOS chip for imaging and the human body communication technology for transmission of images.

Most of the available literature on SBVCE is confined to PillCam. There are very little data on the EndoCapsule, MiroCam, OMOM, and Sayaka in the literature.[4–8] Technical characteristics of the capsules are described in **Table 1**.

AGILE PATENCY CAPSULE

SBVCE is contraindicated for patients with known or suspected small-bowel strictures because of the risk of capsule retention and impaction that may necessitate removal either endoscopically or surgically. Screening fluoroscopic procedures, such as small bowel enteroclysis and small bowel follow-through, are associated with high doses of radiation and false-negative results.

The Agile Patency Capsule (Given Imaging) is a disintegrating, time-controlled capsule developed to identify patients with strictures that may cause retention of the video capsule. This capsule was approved by the FDA in 2006. It consists of a disintegrating capsule with an RF identification tag (RFID) and an RFID scanner.

The Agile Patency Capsule is of the same size as the SBVCE. It has cellophane walls that are filled with lactose (mixed with barium) and surround an RFID. When retained in

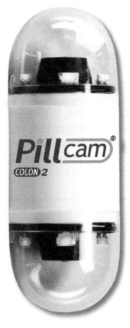

Fig. 1. New PillCam Colon 2 capsule.

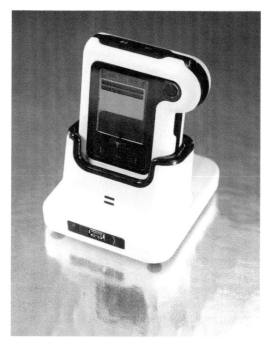

Fig. 2. New PillCam Colon 2 capsule data recorder.

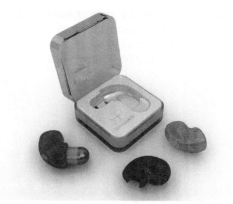

Fig. 3. Mirocam capsule.

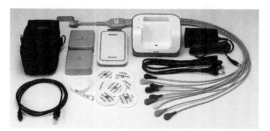

Fig. 4. Mirocam full system.

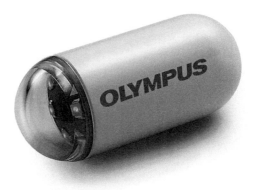

Fig. 5. Olympus endocapsule.

a fluid-filled environment, the core of the patency capsule dissolves after approximately 40 hours, allowing the insoluble outer membrane to collapse and pass. The physician determines the presence of the patency capsule in the body of the patient using the scanner. The Agile Patency Capsule is expected to eliminate the risk of capsule retention in patients with known intestinal strictures who undergo capsule endoscopy.[9]

SB PREPARATION BEFORE SBVCE

The optimal SB preparation for SBVCE is an area of debate in the literature. Manufacturers of capsule endoscopy systems recommend only a clear liquid diet and an 8-hour fast. Several investigators have studied the effect of bowel preparation using polyethylene glycol (PEG) or sodium phosphate on SB visualization.[10]However, the results of

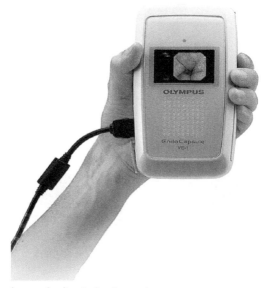

Fig. 6. Olympus endocapsule direct viewing system.

Table 1
Differences between commercially available capsules

	PillCam Colon	PillCam ESO	PillCam SB2	EndoCapsule	MiroCam	OMOM	Sayaka
Length (mm)	26	26	26	26	24	27.9	NA
Weight (g)	3.4	3.4	3.4	3.8	3.4	6	NA
Number of cameras	2	2	1	1	1	1	NA
Frames (per second)	4–35	18	2	2	3	2	NA
Image sensor	CMOS	CMOS	CMOS	CCD	CCD	CCD	NA
Battery life (h)	8	8	8	9	11	8	NA
Antennas	8	3	8	8	9	14	NA
Sleeping mode	Yes	No	No	No	No	No	NA

Abbreviations: CMOS, complementary metal oxide semiconductor; NA, not applicable.

these studies have been contradictory. Some studies reported that bowel preparation resulted in an improvement in visualization, whereas others found no differences in SB visualization or diagnostic yield.[11] A recent meta-analysis has shown that small bowel purgative preparation (PEG solution or sodium phosphate) improves the diagnostic yield of the examination.[12] Another meta-analysis and a systematic review (presented as an abstract) that examined the effectiveness of bowel preparation for VCE also included studies using prokinetics and simethicone (in contrast to the previous study) and showed that bowel preparation had no effect on VCE diagnostic yield.[13] Although adverse events and patient intolerance might be associated with the use of bowel purge for VCE, as inferred from colonoscopy studies, these have not yet been reported.[14]

A new cleansing score system for SB preparation assessing 2 visual parameters was recently published: (1) proportion of visualized mucosa (4-step scale ranging from 0 to 3: score 3, >75%; score 2, 50%–75%; score 1, 25%–50%; score 0, <25%) and (2) degree of obscuration (4-step scale ranging from 0 to 3: score 3, <5% [no obscuration]; score 2, 5%–25% [mild obscuration]; score 1, 25%–50% [moderate obscuration]; score 0, >50% [severe obscuration]).[15]

There is no consensus about the necessity of intestinal preparation for capsule endoscopy, and it should be interesting to develop adequate guidelines to improve its efficacy and tolerability.[16]

INDICATIONS FOR SBVCE

A recent systematic review of 227 original English-language articles involving 22,840 procedures showed that obscure gastrointestinal bleeding (OGIB) is the most common indication (66%) for SBVCE, followed by "clinical symptoms" (10%), definite or suspected Crohn disease (CD) (10%), and other indications (34%).[1]

OGIB

An OGIB is considered in patients with a digestive bleeding when the source of the bleeding remains unexplained after routine endoscopic procedures, including upper gastrointestinal (GI) endoscopy and colonoscopy and more frequently SB imaging modalities.[17] OGIB represents about 5% of all GI bleeding.[18] An overt OGIB with melena or hematochezia must be distinguished from occult digestive bleeding that is characterized by iron-deficient anemia with positive fecal occult blood test

(FOBT) result. Digestive bleeding is now classified as upper GI bleeding, mid-GI bleeding, and lower GI bleeding.[19]

The most common causes of OGIB are located in the SB and are considered as mid-GI bleeding. Nevertheless, 10% to 15% of the so-called OGIB is because of missed lesions located either in the upper GI tract or in the colon.[20] Arteriovenous malformations or angioectasias account for most of the lesions, followed by SB tumors, drug-related lesions, and CD.[18,21]

Several factors have been identified for selecting patients with OGIB in whom the risk of detecting a lesion is high: a serum hemoglobin level less than 10 g/dL, an ongoing overt bleeding (within 15 days), the presence of anemia or recurrent bleeding for more than 6 months, the occurrence of more than 1 episode of bleeding, the coexistence of renal insufficiency, and an occult bleeding with continuous positive FOBT results.[18,19,21–23]

Should all patients with an OGIB be investigated? The American Gastroenterology Association Institute stated that "some patients with OGIB are managed clinically with intermittent blood transfusion along with other non specific supportive measures such as avoidance of anticoagulants as well as oral iron supplementation."[22] In clinical practice, the evaluation of OGIB is a function of the extent of the bleeding and the age of the patient.

Since the last 10 years, several endoscopic methods are available for examining the SB; these methods are either noninvasive, such as the SBVCE, or invasive, such as the assisted-device enteroscopy.[17–19] Several comparative studies that have been compiled in the meta-analysis have demonstrated that SBVCE is superior to push enteroscopy for detecting small-bowel lesions in the case of OGIB.[24,25] Some studies suggest that the double-balloon method has a diagnostic yield similar to that of SBVCE but is obviously more invasive.[26,27] The diagnostic accuracy of SBVCE by obtaining a final diagnosis at 1 year has a negative predictive value close to 100%.[27–29]

Besides the diagnostic accuracy of SBVCE in OGIB, it is mandatory to determine the therapeutic effect of this investigation. Several studies reported a therapeutic effect in 33% to 66% of the patients.[30,31] In a well-designed protocol comparing push enteroscopy with SBVCE as the first-line strategy, De Leusse and colleagues[32] showed that SBVCE has a therapeutic effect (43%) superior to that of push enteroscopy (34%), with less additional procedures.

Is there a role for a second-look SBVCE or other modalities after a nondiagnostic SBVCE first test? The rebleeding rate after a normal SBVCE is very low.[33,34] However, if the rebleeding presentation changes from occult to overt or if the hemoglobin value decreases more than 4 g/dL, there is a need for further investigation. It has been reported that gross abnormalities, including tumors, may be missed by SBVCE, especially in the proximal jejunum.[35]

Long-term follow-up in patients with OGIB showed an 11% to 33% total recurrent bleeding.[18,19] In the case of positive results in SBVCE and subsequent therapeutic enteroscopy, there was 80% no rebleeding.[30] However, Laine and colleagues[36] recently reported a prospective study that enrolled 135 patients with OGIB and a negative workup, including upper GI endoscopy, colonoscopy, and push enteroscopy. These patients were randomized to undergo either SBVCE or SB contrast radiography with a follow-up of 12 months. The diagnostic yields for SBVCE and the SB radiography were 30% and 5%, respectively. However, there was 30% further bleeding in the SBVCE group and 24% in the SB radiography group (no statistical difference).

In conclusion, SBVCE has an excellent diagnostic yield in OGIB, reaching 50% to 60%; it is well admitted that SBVCE should be the first-line procedure in OGIB. If the SBVCE result is negative, the risk of rebleeding is low, but the patient's characteristics and bleeding features should be further investigated.

CD

CD is an inflammatory bowel disease (IBD) that can affect the entire GI tract, with the SB being the most commonly affected site. It is the only site involved in 30% of the cases and, therefore, is difficult to diagnose. Symptoms of CD are heterogeneous but include diarrhea for more than 6 months, abdominal pain, or weight loss. Systemic symptoms of malaise, anorexia, or fever are common. A single gold standard for the diagnosis of CD is not available. The diagnosis is confirmed by clinical evaluation and a combination of endoscopic, histologic, radiologic, or biochemical investigations.[37]

For suspected CD, ileocolonoscopy and biopsies from the terminal ileum and each colonic segment to look for microscopic evidence are first line to establish the diagnosis. The advent of VCE, along with device-assisted enteroscopy (push, single and double balloon, and spiral), has revolutionized SB imaging and has major implications for diagnosis, classification, and therapeutic decision making. A position paper reached by a group of experts in endoscopy and IBD, endorsed by the European Crohn Colitis Organisation and the World Organisation of Digestive Endoscopy, has recently been published.[38] The working parties performed a systematic literature search of their topic with the appropriate keywords using Medline/PubMed/EMBASE and the Cochrane database. The evidence level was graded according to the system of the Oxford Center for Evidence-Based Medicine.

In patients with suspected CD, ileocolonoscopy must be performed before SBVCE. Moreover, SB cross-sectional imaging should generally precede SBVCE. SBVCE is likely to identify mucosal lesions that are compatible with CD in some patients in whom conventional endoscopic and small bowel radiographic imaging modalities have been nondiagnostic, but the diagnosis of CD should not be based on the appearance at the capsule endoscopy alone. Indeed, there is a lack of validated diagnostic criteria for SBVCE for the diagnosis of CD. Endoscopic differentiation of small bowel CD from drug-induced lesions or other diseases is unreliable.

However, SBVCE is better than small bowel follow-through enteroclysis, computed tomography (CT)/magnetic resonance enterography, or enteroclysis for detecting mucosal lesions related to CD.[39,40] A normal SBVCE result has a very high negative predictive value, essentially ruling out SB CD.[41] However, the use of SBVCE is limited by a lack of specificity when SB CD is suspected. Indeed, more than 10% of healthy subjects demonstrate mucosal breaks and erosions in their SB.

In patients with established CD, the role of SBVCE is to focus on the unexplained symptoms when other investigations are inconclusive, if it will alter management. In these patients, the risk of SBVCE retention is increased, particularly in those with known intestinal stenosis. The Agile Patency Capsule reduces the risk of retention.[42] For the assessment of postoperative recurrence of CD, SBVCE should be considered only if ileocolonoscopy is contraindicated or unsuccessful.[37]

In patients with indefinite IBD, SBVCE is helpful in identifying mucosal lesions related to CD. A negative SBVCE result does not exclude a future diagnosis of CD. In a recent report, it has been confirmed that preoperative wireless capsule endoscopy does not predict the outcome after ileal pouch anastomosis.[43]

SBVCE can be safely used in selected children[38] who are even younger than 8 years.[44]

In conclusion, SBVCE should be reserved for patients in whom the clinical suspicion for CD remains high despite negative results with ileocolonoscopy and radiologic examinations.

Other Indications for SBVCE

SB tumors

In patients with SB tumors, the most common indication for SBVCE is an obscure bleeding; in patients who underwent SBVCE for various reasons, the incidence of SB tumors ranged from 2% to 9%.[16,45] SBVCE has good sensitivity in diagnosing malignant tumors as adenocarcinomas, lymphomas, carcinoids, sarcomas, and hamartomas.[46–48] SBVCE also plays a role in identifying benign tumors as GI stromal tumors (**Fig. 7**).[49] Tumors are located in the jejunum (40%–60%), the ileum (25%–40%), and less frequently in the duodenum (15%–20%).[16]

Celiac diseases

Although SBVCE has good sensitivity and specificity for detecting mucosal atrophy, the procedure has limited application in patients with suspected celiac disease[50,51] because a biopsy specimen is needed to confirm the diagnosis; SBVCE is probably more useful in selected cases with refractory or complicated celiac disease.[52]

Hereditary polyposis syndromes

It has been shown that SBVCE is better for diagnosis and surveillance of SB polyps than for that of SB enteroclysis[53]; however, magnetic resonance imaging provides a better estimation of the site and size of the polyps.[54] Although SBVCE is recommended for searching for SB polyps in patients with familial adenomatous polyposis who have duodenal lesions, endoscopy, mainly with a side-view duodenoscope, is preferable to examine the duodenum, especially the ampullary region. SBVCE should be considered as the first-line screening modality for surveillance in patients with Peutz-Jeghers syndrome.[16]

COLON CAPSULE ENDOSCOPY

Colorectal cancer (CRC) is the second leading cause of cancer-related deaths in the Western world. Most of the cases of CRC are believed to arise from adenomatous polyps that progress over the course of many years to invasive adenocarcinoma.[55] Current evidence-based guidelines recommend the screening of average-risk adults, because the early detection and removal of adenomatous polyps has been shown to reduce the incidence of CRC and CRC-related mortality.[56,57] Such screening can reduce CRC incidence and mortality, but effectiveness depends on its quality, ease of use, and patient adherence.[56,58,59]

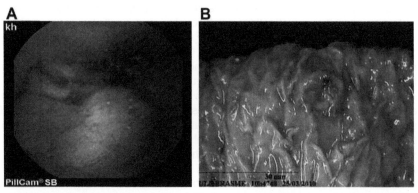

Fig. 7. (A) Capsule endoscopic image and (B) the corresponding macroscopic image of a GI stromal tumor in the terminal ileum.

a mean age of 50 years (range, 18–57 years). In this study, the sensitivities for detecting polyps 6 or 10 mm were 89% and 88%, respectively, with specificities of 76% and 89%, respectively.

The 2 pilot studies and the large multicenter trial that were performed with the PCCE 1 comparing the accuracy of PCCE with that of conventional colonoscopy for detecting colon polyps and cancer have shown that CCE is feasible and safe.[63–65] However, the sensitivity of PCCE for detecting polyps is lower than that of OC. The sensitivity of PCCE significantly increased in the group of patients with a good to excellent preparation.

The sensitivity for detecting polyps that was obtained with PCCE 2 is significantly improved, mainly because of the technical adaptation of the PCCE 2; indeed, the percentage of good to excellent colon cleanliness was similar to that in previous studies than in previous studies.

Two recent meta-analyses including more than 600 patients showed a sensitivity of about 69% and a specificity of about 86%.[67,68]

Although PCCE cannot yet be recommended as a screening procedure for CRC, data are encouraging. This method is minimally invasive and safe and can be performed on an ambulatory basis. Clinical studies provide data to support the potential role of PCCE in the armamentarium of techniques aiming to visualize colon polyps and CRCs. Capsule colonoscopy may be proposed as an alternative for patients unwilling to undergo OC or for those in whom OC was incomplete or contraindicated.[16] Improvements in the definition of the best colon preparation regimen are eagerly expected, as well as studies comparing PCCE with OC and CT colonography in average-risk screening populations. If further improved, capsule colonoscopy may have the potential for dramatically increasing population compliance to CRC screening by offering a minimally invasive screening method for polyps and cancers, which could be performed outside of typical medical offices, potentially in an at-home setting, with the goal of "liberating" medical resources in gastroenterology for the performance of therapeutic endoscopic examinations. Several protocols with the second-generation PCCE 2 are ongoing.

What Could Be the Future for the Colon Capsule?

The future use of PCCE as a tool for exploring the colon, especially as a screening procedure, depends on several factors: (1) Technologic improvement of the capsule: the PCCE 2 already showed significant higher specificity than the PCCE 1. Efforts should be made to lower the reading time. (2) Colon preparation should be improved and simplified to increase the sensitivity of the method, as well as the acceptance rate of the population. (3) Selection of patients based on indication and compliance. Besides CRC screening, PCCE could also be used in patients with IBDs for assessing mucosal healing or postoperative recurrence. (4) Cost should be competitive in comparison to other screening methods.

FUTURE OF VCE

One of the biggest limitations of VCE is the lack of control of navigation. The movement of the capsule is passive because it proceeds by visceral peristalsis and gravity. Therefore, some portions of the GI surface are unlikely to be visualized. The likelihood of missing diagnostically relevant information increases as the lumen size and/or the transit speed increases.

The ability to manipulate the capsule remotely inside the GI tract might be an advantage. Diagnostic accuracy might be improved if more images of the abnormalities or images at different angles or distances are available for examination and if some of

the diagnostic difficulties caused by rapid or slow peristalsis could be overcome. Therapeutic options, cytology, and biopsy might become feasible if remote manipulation were possible.[3]

FUJI INTELLIGENT CHROMO ENDOSCOPY

In addition to the improvement in the chip technology and image quality, Given Imaging introduced a new imaging capability, Fuji Intelligent Chromo Endoscopy (FICE), with PillCam capsule endoscopy system assisted by the Fujinon intelligent color enhancement system (Fujinon, Saitama City, Saitama, Japan).

FICE is a new, virtual chromoendoscopic technique that enhances mucosal visibility, wherein the bandwidth of the conventional endoscopic image is narrowed down arithmetically using computerized spectral estimation technology. There are limited data regarding the use of FICE for SB lesions.[69] A recent retrospective study investigated 40 SBVCE examinations for OGIB (PillCam SB2) and showed that the sensitivity and specificity were 0.90 and 0.55 for FICE and 0.86 and 0.78 for white light imaging, respectively. Significantly more nonsignificant lesions were diagnosed when FICE was used as compared with white light imaging (24, 4; $P<.01$) (**Figs. 8** and **9**).[70]

REMOTE MANIPULATION (CONTROLLED MOTION)

The first study in humans tested a new magnetic maneuverable wireless capsule in a volunteer (as part of a European FP6 project, NEMO [Nano-based capsule-Endoscopy with Molecular imaging and Optical biopsy]). A wireless capsule based on a colon type (Given Imaging) was modified to include neodymium-iron-boron magnets. The capsule's magnetic switch was replaced with a thermal switch and turned on by placing in hot water. One imager was removed from the PillCam colon-based capsule, and the available space was used to house the magnets. A handheld external magnet was used to manipulate this capsule in the esophagus and stomach. Capsule images were viewed on a real-time viewer. The capsule was easily turned and angulated at the cardioesophageal junction. Spinning of the capsule was easily obtained in the stomach.[71] A magnetic internal mechanism with robotic control of the wireless

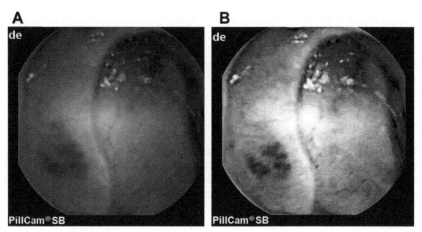

Fig. 8. (*A*) White light image and (*B*) FICE image of a pathologic vascular lesion using RAPID 6 system.

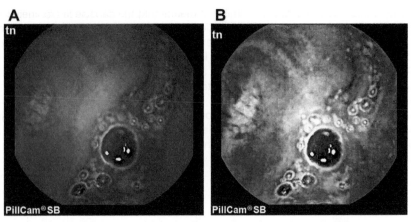

Fig. 9. (*A*) White light image and (*B*) FICE image of an ulcer using RAPID 6 system.

endoscopic capsule has recently been described, which could strongly improve the use of the wireless video capsule (**Fig. 10**).[72,73]

POWER MANAGEMENT (BATTERYLESS POWER)

The idea of wireless battery power has been considered, whereby the power for the capsule is supplied from an external source and sent wirelessly to the capsule.

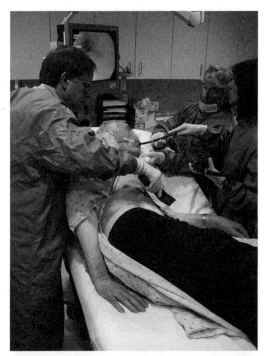

Fig. 10. Remote magnetic manipulation. (*From* Swain P, Toor A, Volke F, et al. Remote magnetic manipulation of a wireless capsule endoscope in the esophagus and stomach of humans (with videos). Gastrointest Endosc 2010. 71:1290-3; with permission.)

The use of this wireless power transmission means that the capsule is not limited by the battery lifetime and the image acquisition is not limited to 2 images per second.

RF SYSTEM lab has developed a batteryless capsule. The Norika3 capsule was introduced in 2001 and is 9 to 23 mm in length. The capsule has not yet achieved FDA clearance. One publication describes a capsule with a CCD imager for acquiring images, with a focus adjustment and rotation mechanism; the capsule moves by peristalsis.[74]

Also, Olympus (Tokyo, Japan) has introduced a batteryless capsule with in vivo capabilities such as drug delivery, controlled motion, and ultrasound scanning.[75]

No clinical trials have yet been published for any clinical use of both of these capsules.[76]

DRUG DELIVERY CAPSULE

Two new capsules, the IntelliSite (Innovative Devices, Raleigh, NC, USA) and Enterion (Phaeton Research, Nottingham, UK), have some promising tools for collecting absorption data in the GI tract and can be used for targeted drug delivery.[77]

MICROBIOPSY CAPSULE

Pilot data from centers developing diagnostic and therapeutic capsules have demonstrated the feasibility of performing mucosal biopsies using a spring-loaded Crosby capsule–type device guided by real-time imaging capability and RF-controlled remote manipulation or a rotational microbiopsy device consisting of a trigger with a paraffin block and a rotational tissue-cutting razor with a torsion controller designed to operate sequentially so that tissue sampling, sealing, and fixing are achieved in single operation. The Versatile Endoscopic Capsule for gastrointestinal TumOr Recognition and therapy (VECTOR) project, funded by the European Commission, is developing a minirobot endowed with actuation modules, mechanisms, sensors, embedded controls, and human-machine interface to navigate and intervene in the GI tract for early detection.[78]

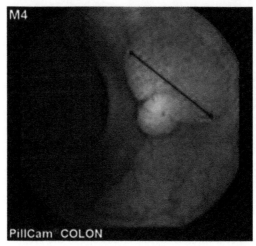

Fig. 11. Measurement capability of Colon 2 capsule with RAPID 6 system for colonic polyps.

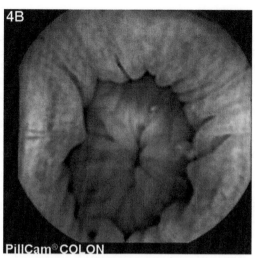

Fig. 12. Picture showing normal transverse colon using PillCam Colon 2 capsule.

THE NEW GENERATION OF PILLCAM COLON 2

The features of this new colon capsule (PCCE 2) have been described earlier. Briefly, this capsule has an integrated LCD with a regimen reminder system. The "Gastric passage" algorithm detects when the capsule has left the stomach. At this stage, the patient is reminded to take the first boost of Phospho-Soda and the capsule goes into alternative frame rendering mode. Therefore the need for real-time reviewing is eliminated. The capsule works in an ultralow frame rate (power conservation mode) while in the stomach. The PCCE 2 has the advantages of saving batteries, automatically indicating the passage of the pylorus, and increasing the number of images when moving. Moreover, the software is equipped with a system that allows assessing the size of the polyps (**Figs. 11–13**).

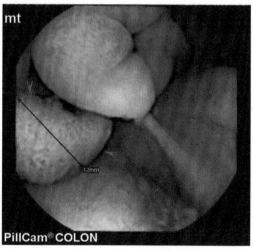

Fig. 13. Picture showing large sessile polyp in front of the ileocecal valve using PillCam Colon 2 capsule.

SUMMARY

VCE is a recent and noninvasive technology that extended endoscopy, stimulated research, and was rapidly integrated in clinical practice. SBVCE is now recognized as the first-line procedure in obscure OGIB, but the procedure has many other indications also. The development of the colon capsule opens a new era for wireless endoscopy and is promising for screening of CRC and IBDs. Recent data have shown that the second generation of the colon capsule significantly increased the sensitivity for detecting colonic polyps. There already exists inventive technologic adaptations such as the remote control system, batteryless capsule, and adapted chromoendoscopy. Research on the therapeutic capabilities of VCE is in progress.

REFERENCES

1. Zhuan L, Rui G, Can X, et al. Indications and detection, completion, and retention rates of small-bowel capsule endoscopy: a systematic review. Gastrointest Endosc 2010;71:280–6.
2. Waterman M, Eliakim R. Capsule enteroscopy of the small intestine. Abdom Imaging 2009;34:452–8.
3. Swain P. The future of wireless capsule endoscopy. World J Gastroenterol 2008; 14:4142–5.
4. Bang S, Park JY, Jeong S, et al. First clinical trial of the "MiRo" capsule endoscope by using a novel transmission technology: electric-field propagation. Gastrointest Endosc 2009;69:253–9.
5. Kim HM, Kim YJ, Kim HJ, et al. A pilot study of sequential capsule endoscopy using MiroCam and Pillcam SB devices with different transmission technologies. Gut Liver 2010;4:192–200.
6. Cave DR, Fleischer DE, Leighton JA, et al. A multicenter randomized comparison of the Endocapsule and the Pillcam SB. Gastrointest Endosc 2008;68:487–94.
7. Hartmann D, Eickhoff A, Damian U, et al. Diagnosis of small-bowel pathology using paired capsule endoscopy with two different devices: a randomized study. Endoscopy 2007;39:1041–5.
8. Gay G, Delvaux M. Small-bowel endoscopy. Endoscopy 2008;40:140–6.
9. Herrerias J, Leighton J, Costamagna G, et al. Agile patency system eliminates risk of capsule retention in patients with known strictures who undergo capsule endoscopy. Gastrointest Endosc 2008;67:902–9.
10. Ben-Soussan E, Savoye G, Antonietti M, et al. Factors that affect gastric passage of video capsule. Gastrointest Endosc 2005;62:785–90.
11. Viazis N, Sgouros S, Papaxoinis K, et al. Bowel preparation increases the diagnostic yield of capsule endoscopy: a prospective, randomized, controlled study. Gastrointest Endosc 2004;60:534–8.
12. Niv Y. Efficiency of bowel preparation for capsule endoscopy examination: a meta-analysis. World J Gastroenterol 2008;14:1313–7.
13. Rokkas T, Papaxoinis K, Triantafyllou K, et al. Does purgative preparation influence the diagnostic yield of small bowel video capsule endoscopy? A meta-analysis. Am J Gastroenterol 2009;104:219–27.
14. Mergener K, Ponchon T, Gralnek I, et al. Literature review and recommendations for clinical application of small-bowel capsule endoscopy, based on a panel discussion by international experts. Consensus statements for small-bowel capsule endoscopy, 2006/2007. Endoscopy 2007;39:895–909.
15. Park SC, Keum B, Hyun JJ, et al. A novel cleansing score system for capsule endoscopy. World J Gastroenterol 2010;16:875–80.

16. Ladas SD, Triantafyllou K, Spada C, et al. European Society of Gastrointestinal Endoscopy (ESGE): recommendations (2009) on clinical use of video capsule endoscopy to investigate small-bowel, esophageal and colonic diseases. Endoscopy 2010;42:220–7.

17. Zuckerman GR, Prakash C, Askin MP, et al. AGA technical review on the evaluation and management of occult and obscure gastrointestinal bleeding. Gastroenterology 2000;118:201–21.

18. Cellier C. Obscure gastrointestinal bleeding: role of video capsule and double-balloon enteroscopy. Best Pract Res Clin Gastroenterol 2008;22:329–40.

19. Gerson LB. Capsule endoscopy and deep enteroscopy: indications for the practicing clinician. Gastroenterology 2009;137:1197–201.

20. Descamps C, Schmit A, Van Gossum A. "Missed" upper gastrointestinal tract lesions may explain "occult" bleeding. Endoscopy 1999;41:2348–52.

21. Van Gossum A. Obscure digestive bleeding. Best Pract Res Clin Gastroenterol 2001;15:155–74.

22. Raju G, Gerson L, Das A, et al. American Gastroenterology Association (AGA) Institute technical review on obscure gastrointestinal bleeding. Gastroenterology 2007;133:1697–717.

23. Carey EJ, Leighton JA, Heigh RI, et al. A single-center experience of 260 consecutive patients undergoing capsule endoscopy for obscure gastrointestinal bleeding. Am J Gastroenterol 2007;102:89–95.

24. Chen X. A meta-analysis of the yield of capsule endoscopy compared to double-balloon enteroscopy in patients with small bowel diseases. World J Gastroenterol 2007;28:4372–8.

25. Triester J, Leighton J, Leontiadis G, et al. A meta-analysis of the yield of capsule endoscopy compared to other diagnostic modalities in patients with obscure gastrointestinal bleeding. Am J Gastroenterol 2005;100:2407–18.

26. Apostolopoulos P, Liatsos C, Gralnek IM, et al. The role of wireless capsule endoscopy in investigating unexplained iron deficiency anemia after negative endoscopic evaluation of the upper and lower gastrointestinal tract. Endoscopy 2006;38:1127–32.

27. Marmo R, Rotondano G, Casetti T, et al. Degree of concordance between double-balloon enteroscopy and capsule endoscopy in obscure gastrointestinal bleeding: a multicenter study. Endoscopy 2009;41:587–92.

28. Pennazio M, Santucci R, Rondonotti E, et al. Outcome of patients with obscure gastrointestinal bleeding after capsule endoscopy: report of 100 consecutive cases. Gastroenterology 2004;126:643–53.

29. Delvaux M, Fassler I, Gay G. Clinical usefulness of the endoscopic video capsule as the initial intestinal investigation in patients with obscure digestive bleeding: validation of a diagnostic strategy based on the patient outcome after 12 months. Endoscopy 2004;36:1067–73.

30. Kaffes A, Siah C, Koo J. Clinical outcomes after double-balloon enteroscopy in patients with obscure GI bleeding and a positive capsule endoscopy. Gastrointest Endosc 2007;66:304–9.

31. Arakawa D, Ohmiya N, Nakamura M, et al. Outcome after enteroscopy for patients with obscure GI bleeding: diagnostic comparison between double-balloon endoscopy and videocapsule endoscopy. Gastrointest Endosc 2009;69:866–74.

32. De Leusse A, Vahedi K, Edery J, et al. Capsule endoscopy or push enteroscopy of first-line exploration of obscure gastrointestinal bleeding. Gastroenterology 2007;132:855–62.

33. Lai L, Wong G, Chow D, et al. Long-term follow-up of patients with obscure gastrointestinal bleeding after negative capsule endoscopy. Am J Gastroenterol 2006;10:1224–8.
34. Viazis N, Papaxoinis K, Vlacho Giannakos J, et al. Is there a role for second-look capsule endoscopy in patients with obscure GI bleeding after a non-diagnostic first test. Gastrointest Endosc 2009;69:850–6.
35. Postgate A, Despott E, Burling D, et al. Significant small-bowel lesions detected by alternative diagnostic modalities after negative capsule endoscopy. Gastrointest Endosc 2008;68:1209–14.
36. Laine L, Sahota A, Shah A, et al. Does capsule endoscopy improve outcomes in obscure gastrointestinal bleeding? Randomized trial versus dedicated small bowel radiography. Gastroenterology 2010;138:1673–80.
37. Van Assche G, Dignass A, Panes J, et al. The second European evidence-based consensus on the diagnosis and management of Crohn's disease: definitions and diagnosis. Journal of Crohn's and Colitis 2010;4:7–27.
38. Bourreille A, Ignjatovic A, Aabakken L, et al. Role of small-bowel endoscopy in the management of patients with inflammatory bowel disease: an international OMED-ECCO consensus. Endoscopy 2009;41:618–37.
39. Triester S, Leighton J, Leontiadis G, et al. A meta-analysis of the yield of capsule endoscopy compared to other diagnostic modalities in patients with non-stricturing small bowel Crohn's disease. Am J Gastroenterol 2006;101:954–64.
40. Dionisio PM, Gurudu SR, Leighton JA, et al. Capsule endoscopy has a significantly higher diagnostic yield in patients with suspected and established small-bowel Crohn's disease: a meta-analysis. Am J Gastroenterol 2010;105:1240–8.
41. Leighton J, Gralnek I, Richner R, et al. Capsule endoscopy in suspected small bowel Crohn's disease: economic impact of disease diagnosis and treatment. World J Gastroenterol 2009;15:5685–92.
42. Mehdizadeh S, Chen G, Barkodar L, et al. Capsule endoscopy in patients with Crohn's disease: diagnostic yield and safety. Gastrointest Endosc 2010;71:121–7.
43. Murrell Z, Vasiliauskas E, Melmed G, et al. Preoperative wireless capsule endoscopy does not predict outcome after ileal pouch-anal anastomosis. Dis Colon Rectum 2010;53:293–300.
44. Fritscher-Ravens A, Siherbakov P, Buffer P, et al. The feasibility of wireless capsule endoscopy in detecting small intestinal pathology in children under the age of 8 years: a multicenter European study. Gut 2009;58:1467–72.
45. Urbain D, De Looze D, Demedts I, et al. Video capsule endoscopy in small-bowel malignancy: a multicenter Belgian study. Endoscopy 2006;38:408–11.
46. Bailey AA, Debinski HS, Appleyard MN, et al. Diagnosis and outcome of small bowel tumors found by capsule endoscopy: a three-center Australian experience. Am J Gastroenterol 2006;101:2237–43.
47. Cobrin GM, Pittman RH, Lewis BS. Increased diagnostic yield of small bowel tumors with capsule endoscopy. Cancer 2006;107:22–7.
48. Estevez E, Gonzalez-Conde B, Vazquez-Iglesias JL, et al. Incidence of tumoral pathology according to study using capsule endoscopy for patients with obscure gastrointestinal bleeding. Surg Endosc 2007;21:1776–80.
49. Rondonotti E, Pennazio M, Toth E, et al. Small-bowel neoplasms in patients undergoing video capsule endoscopy: a multicenter European study. Endoscopy 2008;40:488–95.
50. Rondonotti E, de Franchis R. Diagnosing celiac disease: is the videocapsule a suitable tool? Dig Liver Dis 2007;39:145–7.

51. Rondonotti E, Spada C, Cave D, et al. Video capsule enteroscopy in the diagnosis of celiac disease: a multicenter study. Am J Gastroenterol 2007;102: 1624–31.
52. Daum S, Wahnschaffe U, Glasenapp R, et al. Capsule endoscopy in refractory celiac disease. Endoscopy 2007;39:455–8.
53. Mata A, Llach J, Castells A, et al. A prospective trial comparing wireless capsule endoscopy and barium contrast series for small-bowel surveillance in hereditary GI polyposis syndromes. Gastrointest Endosc 2005;61:721–5.
54. Gupta A, Postgate A, Burling D, et al. A prospective study of MR enterography versus capsule endoscopy for the surveillance of adult patients with the Peutz-Jeghers syndrome. AJR Am J Roentgenol 2010;195:108–16.
55. Bond JH. Clinical evidence for the adenoma-carcinoma sequence, and the management of patients with colorectal adenomas. Semin Gastrointest Dis 2000;11:176–84.
56. Winawer SJ, Zauber AG, Ho MN, et al. Prevention of colorectal cancer by colonoscopic polypectomy. The National Poly Study Workgroup. N Engl J Med 1993; 329:1977–81.
57. Winawer SJ, Zauber AG. The advanced adenoma as the primary target of screening. Gastrointest Endosc Clin N Am 2002;12:1–9.
58. Martinez ME, Baron JA, Lieberman DA, et al. A pooled analysis of advanced colorectal neoplasia diagnoses after colonoscopic polypectomy. Gastroenterology 2009;136:832–41.
59. Levin B, Lieberman DA, McFarland B, et al. Screening and surveillance of the early detection of colorectal cancer and adenomatous polyps, 2008: a joint guideline from the American Cancer Society, the US Multi-Society Task Force on colorectal cancer, and the American College of Radiology. Gastroenterology 2008;134:1570–95.
60. Rex DK, Helbig C. High yields of small and flat adenomas with high-definition colonoscopies using either white light or narrow band imaging. Gastroenterology 2007;133:42–7.
61. Ponchon T. Colon tumors and colonoscopy. Endoscopy 2007;39:992–7.
62. Eliakim R, Yassin K, Niv Y, et al. Prospective multicenter performance evaluation of the second-generation colon capsule compared with colonoscopy. Endoscopy 2009;41:1026–31.
63. Eliakim R, Fireman Z, Gralnek IM, et al. Evaluation of the Pillcam colon capsule in the detection of colonic pathology: results of the first multicenter, prospective, comparative study. Endoscopy 2006;38:963–70.
64. Schoofs N, Devière J, Van Gossum A. Pillcam colon capsule endoscopy compared with colonoscopy for colorectal diagnosis: a prospective pilot study. Endoscopy 2006;38:971–7.
65. Van Gossum A, Navas MM, Fernandez-Urien I, et al. Capsule endoscopy versus colonoscopy for the detection of polyps and cancer. N Engl J Med 2009;361:264–70.
66. Sieg A, Friedrich K, Sieg U. Is Pillcam colon capsule endoscopy ready for colorectal cancer screening? A prospective feasibility study in a community gastroenterology practice. Am J Gastroenterol 2009;104:848–54.
67. Rokkas T, Papaxoinis K, Triantafyllou K, et al. A meta-analysis evaluating the accuracy of colon capsule endoscopy in detecting colon polyps. Gastrointest Endosc 2010;71:792–8.
68. Spada C, Riccioni ME, Hassan C, et al. Pillcam colon capsule endoscopy: a prospective, randomized trial comparing two regimens of preparation. J Clin Gastroenterol 2010 [online].

69. Pohl J, Aschmoneit I, Schuhmann S, et al. Computed image modification for enhancement of small-bowel surface structure at video capsule endoscopy. Endoscopy 2010;42:490–2.
70. Gupta T, Ibrahim M, Deviere J, et al. Is Fujinon Intelligent Color Enhancement (FICE) assisted capsule endoscopy (CE) helpful for analyzing obscure GI bleeding (OGIB)? Gastroenterology 2010;138:S667–8.
71. Swain P, Toor A, Keller J. Remote magnetic manipulation of a wireless capsule endoscope in the esophagus and stomach of humans (with videos). Gastrointest Endosc 2010;71:1290–3.
72. Valdastri D, Quaglia C, Buselli E, et al. A magnetic internal mechanism for precise orientation of the camera in wireless endoluminal applications. Endoscopy 2010; 42:481–6.
73. Ciuti G, Donlin R, Valdastri D, et al. Robotic versus manual control in magnetic steering of an endoscopic capsule. Endoscopy 2010;42:148–52.
74. Uehara A, Hoshina K. Capsule endoscope NORIKA system. Minim Invasive Ther Allied Technol 2003;12:227–34.
75. Kusuda Y. A further step beyond wireless capsule endoscopy. Sensor Rev 2005; 25:259–60.
76. Twomey K, Marchesi J. Swallowable capsule technology: current perspectives and future directions. Endoscopy 2009;11:357–62.
77. Wilding I, Hirst P, Connor A. Development of a new engineering based capsule for human drug absorption studies. Pharm Sci Technol Today 2000;11:385–92.
78. Sharma VK. The future is wireless: advances in wireless diagnostic and therapeutic technologies in gastroenterology. Gastroenterology 2009;137:434–9.

New Options of Cholangioscopy

Grischa Terheggen, MD*, Horst Neuhaus, MD

KEYWORDS

- Cholangioscopy • Bile duct • Peroral cholangioscopy
- Percutaneous transhepatic cholangioscopy

In the evaluation of biliary diseases, cholangioscopy is considered as complementary procedure to radiographic imaging by computed tomography (CT) scan, magnetic resonance imaging (MRI), magnetic resonance cholangiopancreatography (MRCP),[1,2] endoscopic retrograde cholangiopancreatography (ERCP),[3] endoscopic ultrasonography (EUS),[4,5] and intraductal ultrasonography (IDUS).[6,7] Direct visualization of the bile duct is the premier advantage of cholangioscopy over these indirect imaging techniques. Peroral cholangioscopy (POCS) and percutaneous transhepatic cholangioscopy (PTCS) improve accuracy in differentiation between benign and malignant processes, allowing targeted sampling of tissue and precise mapping of tumors in preparation for surgical resection. Moreover, cholangioscopy provides endoscopic guidance for therapeutic interventions, such as electrohydraulic lithotripsy (EHL), laser lithotripsy (LL), photodynamic therapy (PDT), and argon plasma coagulation (APC). However, cholangioscopy has not gained wide acceptance because of several technical limitations such as scope fragility, impaired steerability, limited irrigation, and suction capabilities, as well as the need for two experienced endoscopists. Several recent innovations such as the implementation of electronic video cholangioscopes and the development of single-operator systems, including the semidisposable SpyGlass Direct Visualization System and the direct biliary approach with ultraslim upper endoscopes, facilitate the procedure and promise to increase the diagnostic and therapeutic yield of cholangioscopy.

EQUIPMENT AND TECHNIQUES

POCS was initially described in 1976.[8,9] PTCS was also developed in the 1970s.[10] The adoption of these procedures has been slowed in part by technological limitations of the cholangioscopes. One of the first reports demonstrated a fiberscope of 8.8 mm diameter, which was inserted perorally into the biliary system after endoscopic

This work was not supported by any funding.
The authors have nothing to disclose.
Department of Internal Medicine, Evangelisches Krankenhaus Düsseldorf, Kirchfeldstraße 40, 40217 Düsseldorf, Germany
* Corresponding author.
E-mail address: grischa.terheggen@googlemail.com

sphincterotomy without the need of a second guiding scope.[11] In the following years the idea of guiding a small-caliber "baby" cholangioscope through the channel of a dedicated larger channel "mother" duodenoscope into the common bile duct (CBD) gained wide acceptance. This "mother-baby" system is operated by 2 experienced endoscopists. The conventional fiberoptic scopes used in the mother-baby system have a distal diameter of 4.5 mm.[12,13] The scopes have one instrumental channel and the tip deflection is limited to one plane (up-down) of approximately 90° without lateral deflection. The baby scopes are fragile and their optic fibers are prone to break easily from pressure applied with the elevator of the duodenoscope. These scopes require a dedicated light source, image processor, and water-air pump. Finally the baby scope image is projected onto a separate video monitor. Two endoscopists are required and a prior sphincterotomy or balloon sphincteroplasty is usually necessary to insert the baby scope into the CBD. To facilitate ductal intubation, administration of agents that relax the sphincter of Oddi, such as hyoscines, glucagon, and isosorbide dinitrate, have been reported to be helpful.[14–16] Inserting the baby scope over a guidewire into the duct reduces the need for elevator use and risk of scope damage. Once the scope is advanced to the target location, the guidewire should be removed to permit use of the accessory channel for irrigation and introduction of devices. Several miniscopes have been developed with reduced diameters ranging from 2 to 3.5 mm, allowing insertion thorough conventional therapeutic duodenoscopes and their delivery into even small bile ducts. If the outer diameter is less than 2.5 mm, access without prior sphincterotomy is possible.[17–20] A fine-caliber flexible miniscope created by Soda and colleagues[21,22] allowed access to the CBD without sphincterotomy, due to its external diameter of 2.09 mm including, unlike many other miniscopes, a central working channel of 0.72 mm. Similarly, Sander and Poesl[23] have developed a less fragile, steerable new miniscope for peroral cholangioscopy with 2 different degrees of stiffness and 2 channels: a 0.4-mm (1.2F) irrigation channel and a 1.2-mm (3.6F) working channel through which a probe for EHL and a stone extraction basket can be passed. Slightly larger miniscopes with bidirectional angulation systems and instrumental channels were developed by several companies.[24] Despite these advances, POCS has remained a very cumbersome and time-consuming procedure that has not reached the expected popularity because it requires 2 experienced endoscopists to perform and has a small spectrum of possible applications.[25] However, image quality and size have been significantly improved by the implementation of video cholangioscopes that use high-resolution video chips (**Fig. 1**).[26–28] The charge-coupled device (CCD) video chip is mounted in the distal tip of the scope and provides a 100° forward direction field of view. Disadvantages of these scopes were the lack of an accessory channel for interventional applications or a very limited working channel of only 0.5 mm. A newer "hybrid" video baby scope integrates a 1.2-mm accessory channel into a scope of 2.8 mm external diameter.[29] The CCD unit is located in the control section, which protects the video chip from the usual scope trauma and may improve the durability of the scope. The image quality of glass fiber–based hybrid cholangioscopes with the CCD unit located in the control section is inferior to those with the CCD unit located in the tip of the scope.[30] However, the video cholangioscope is still fragile and is not yet widely available. Despite technological advances in the design and maneuverability of miniature endoscopes and their accessories, few technical improvements have been made regarding the main concept of the mother-baby system. Limited tip deflection and the lack of optimal irrigation systems compromise visibility, requiring extra time and effort to complete the procedure.[14,31] An additional limitation is the small caliber (range 0.5–1.2 mm) of the working channel that allows the use of only small biopsy

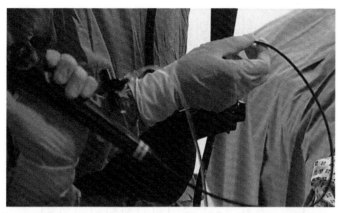

Fig. 1. Mother-and-baby cholangioscopy. The tube of the video cholangioscope is inserted into the working channel of a therapeutic duodenoscope, which is attached to a special belt ("scope dock device") of the endoscopist to facilitate the procedure.

forceps, which are able to obtain very small and often inadequate tissue samples. **Table 1** summarizes and compares the currently available cholangioscopic technologies.[14]

The search for a less cumbersome technique has led to the application of ultraslim gastroscopes to perform direct visualization and treatment of biliary disease.[32] With external diameters of 5 to 6 mm, these instruments are only suitable for examination of the CBD after a sphincterotomy. An ERCP is performed first to place a 0.035-in diameter super-stiff guidewire as far into the bile duct as possible. After sphincterotomy the duodenoscope is cautiously removed and the ultraslim upper endoscope is then inserted over the guidewire, under fluoroscopic and endoscopic control, into the duodenum and across the ampulla of Vater into the CBD. Even with the guidewire in place, intubation and deep advancement of the endoscope into the bile duct can be limited by vector forces that tend to advance the scope along the axis of the duodenum, as well as looping the scope in the stomach.[30,32] Loop formation can be reduced by use of an overtube, which can be mounted on the gastroscope, to facilitate this part of the procedure. Although the currently available overtube is too large in diameter for an ultraslim endoscope, making it difficult to manipulate both the overtube and the endoscope, it has been frequently adopted among Japanese and Korean endoscopists during POCS with ultraslim upper endoscopes.[33] A pilot study evaluated the feasibility of POCS with an ultraslim endoscope and an intraductal balloon that can be anchored in a branch of an intrahepatic duct (IHD) with the similar procedure using a guidewire.[34] A specialized 5F balloon catheter is required to fit the 2.0-mm working channel of the endoscope. After anchoring the intraductal balloon within a biliary branch, the endoscope can be advanced over the balloon catheter into the proximal biliary system. The investigators reported a success rate of 95.2% intraductal balloon-guided POCS compared with 45.5% for wire-guided POCS, and described no difficulties in negotiating through the hilum into the right or left ductal system once they were in the CBD. In addition, repeated advancement and withdrawal of the scope through the firmly anchored balloon catheter was possible. Nevertheless, anchoring the balloon within a branch of the IHD is not possible in some patients, and the intraductal balloon should be withdrawn from the scope to perform tissue sampling or therapeutic intervention, which can create technical difficulties in maintaining the desired endoscope position.[34] An ultrathin balloon catheter was recently

Table 1
Details of cholangioscopic systems

	Distal Diameter (mm)	Accessory Channel (mm)	Working Length (cm)	Angulation (up/down/left/right)	Field of View	Route
Olympus						
CHF-BP30 (fiberoptic)	3.4	1.2	187	160°/130°/–/–	90°	POCS
CHF-BP160 (video)	2.9	0.5	200	90°/90°/–/–	90°	POCS
CHF-BP160F (fiberoptic + video)	2.8	1.2	200	70°/70°/–/–	90°	POCS
CHF-CB30 (fiberoptic)	2.7	1.2	45–70	120°/120°/–/–	75°	PTCS
Pentax						
FCP-8P (fiberoptic)	2.8	0.75	190	90°/90°/–/–	90°	POCS
FCP-9P (fiberoptic)	3.1	1.2	190	90°/90°/–/–	90°	POCS
FCN-15X (fiberoptic)	4.8	2.2	35	180°/130°/–/–	125°	PTCS
Boston Scientific						
SpyGlass probe	0.77		300	30°/30°	70°	POCS
SpyScope catheter (4 lm)	3.3 (10F)	1.2 + 0.6/0.6	220	30°/30°		

developed for placement over a guidewire by means of standard ERCP. After inflation and anchoring in the proximal biliary tree the balloon can be sealed before detachment of the handle. This technique allows removal of the duodenoscope and backloading of an ultraslim gastroscope for subsequent insertion over the anchored balloon catheter. The catheter can then be removed for insertion of accessories such as biopsy forceps (**Fig. 2**A–D). This promising new method is currently under clinical evaluation.

POCS with ultraslim endoscopes offers advantages such as performance by a single operator and superior image quality of the ductal mucosa. Furthermore, high-definition imaging and narrow-band imaging (NBI) can be obtained, which leads to a better visualization of neoplastic lesions.[35] The separate water and air channels improve intraductal visualization and the 2.0-mm working channel allows the passage of larger biopsy forceps, which may increase the diagnostic yield during tissue sampling. Moreover, the working channel enables therapeutic interventions including EHL, LL, tissue ablation, and direct stent placement. **Table 2** summarizes and compares the currently available ultraslim endoscopes used for cholangioscopy.[36]

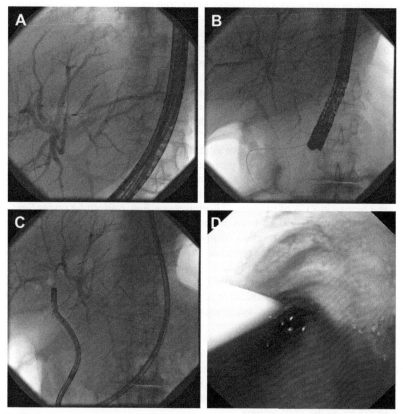

Fig. 2. (*A*) A specially designed anchoring balloon is inflated in the left hepatic duct by means of an ERCP in a patient with suspected hilar cholangiocarcinoma. (*B*) After detachment of the handle of the catheter the duodenoscope is removed, leaving the anchored inflated balloon in place. (*C*) An ultraslim gastroscope is advanced through the papilla toward the hilum after backloading over the anchored balloon catheter. (*D*) Endoscopic visualization of the hilum showing the balloon catheter entering the left hepatic duct.

Table 2
Details of ultraslim upper endoscopes for cholangioscopy

	Distal Diameter (mm)	Accessory Channel (mm)	Working Length (cm)	Angulation (up/down)	Angulation (left/right)	Field of View
Olympus						
GIF-N230	6	2	92.5	180°/180°	160°/160°	120°
GIF-XP 160	5.9	2	103	210°/90°	100°/100°	120°
GIF-XP 180 N	5.5	2	110	210°/90°	100°/100°	120°
Pentax						
FG-16 V	5.3	2	92.5	180°/180°	160°/160°	125°
Fujinon						
EG-530 N	5.9	2	110	210°/90°	100°/100°	120°

POCS with the mother-baby system can be performed by a single endoscopist with the help of a baby scope–holding breastplate.[37] This technique has been reported to be successful in management of patients with choledocholithiasis. The recently introduced SpyGlass Direct Visualization System is designed for single-operator examination as well.[38] This system can be strapped to the duodenoscope just below the operating channel with a silastic belt. The modular system consists of 3 components: (1) a reusable 0.77-mm diameter 6000-pixel fiber-optical probe (SpyGlass) for direct visual examination of the targeted bile duct; (2) a 10F disposable 4-lm catheter (SpyScope) consisting of a 0.9-mm channel for the optical probe, a 1.2-mm instrumentation channel, and 2 dedicated 0.6-mm irrigation channels; (3) a disposable 3F biopsy forceps (SpyBite) for tissue acquisition in the biliary system. The catheter has 4-way tip deflection (each more than 30°), which improves the maneuverability of the catheter in the duct and allows intubation of individual intrahepatic branches (**Fig. 3**A–C). An initial feasibility study demonstrated procedural success in 32 of 35 patients (91%) with indeterminate biliary strictures, with 71% sensitivity and 100% specificity in differentiating malignant versus benign pathologies and lesion-directed successful biopsy in 71% of patients.[39] Furthermore, EHL performed under SpyGlass guidance cleared the bile duct from stones in all patients (5/5) after failure of prior conventional ERCP stone extraction. These results were confirmed by a prospective international multicenter registry reporting on 297 patients with either diagnostic or therapeutic indications in biliary disease. The study demonstrated an overall procedural success rate of 89% with a sensitivity of SpyGlass visual impression in diagnosing malignancy of 88%. Adequate stone visualization and initiation of stone fragmentation and removal was successful in 92%.[40] Although the image quality is inferior to CCD chip cholangioscopes, visualization is enhanced by the 4-way deflected steering of the SpyGlass tip, which allows unrestricted access to all bile duct quadrants and the possibility of ample continuous irrigation to keep the field of view clear of blood, stone debris, sludge, or pus during visual inspection and biopsy. Therefore, direct visualization for the evaluation of biliary disease or therapy for biliary stones with the SpyGlass system can broaden the cholangioscopic options in diagnostic and therapeutic applications.

If the less invasive peroral route is not feasible or fails, PTCS can be performed by a single endoscopist along with an assistant for diagnostic and therapeutic interventions such as insertion of biopsy forceps or probes for lithotripsy. A sequential establishment of an appropriate cutaneobiliary fistula ("sinus tract") is probably safer than a one-step approach. After MRCP-guided selection of the site of interest and selection

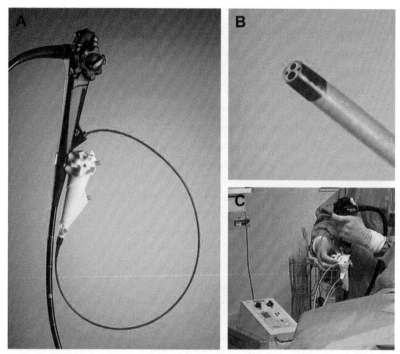

Fig. 3. (*A*) SpyGlass access and delivery catheter inserted though the instrumentation channel of a therapeutic duodenoscope; the proximal instrumentation part of the device is attached to the tube of the duodenoscope, which allows its use by a single endoscopist. (*B*) The SpyGlass Direct Visualization System is used for intraductal laser lithotripsy under direct visual control. (*C*) The green laser light is transmitted from the generator via an ultra-thin glass fiber inserted through the accessory channel of the catheter.

of the most appropriate biliary segment, a percutaneous transhepatic catheter is placed. This tract can then be dilated every 2 or 3 days leaving larger drainage catheters in place up to a diameter of 16 French. This approach allows establishment of a mature tract within 8 to 10 days. A cholangioscope or bronchoscope can then be advanced into the biliary tree without need of a sheath. The tract predetermines the ducts that can be accessed with the cholangioscope; maneuvering to the opposite liver segment may be impossible through a single percutaneous tract.[41] Cholangioscopes designed for percutaneous use have larger accessory channels and are accompanied by a broader array of therapeutic devices. The shorter working length and distance to the target area improve the ability to torque the scope for 4-quadrant visualization.

DIAGNOSTIC APPLICATIONS

The diagnostic indications for peroral cholangioscopy (POCS) including the evaluation of biliary strictures or intraductal filling defects are listed in **Box 1**. PTCS is considered when transpapillary procedures fail because of inaccessibility of the papilla of Vater owing to previous surgery, difficult duodenal diverticulum, inaccessibility of a biliodigestive anastomosis, for example, hepaticojejunostomy, or nonpassable and not adequately dilatable bile duct strictures.

Box 1
Diagnostic indications of cholangioscopy

Visual characterization and optically guided biopsy of biliary strictures

    Indeterminate strictures

    Dominant strictures in primary sclerosing cholangitis (PSC)

Evaluation of fixed ductal filling defects noted on cholangiography or other imaging

Differentiation of benign versus malignant intraductal mass

    Improved yield of tissue sampling under visual guidance

    Enhanced image by use of chromocholangioscopy with dye solution, autofluorescence imaging (AFI), and NBI

Precise mapping and delineation of intraductal tumor spread before resection

Collection of significant fluid sample for cytology

Visual evaluation of intraductal spread of ampullary adenoma

Visual evaluation of choledochal cyst

Visual evaluation for ductal ischemia after liver transplant

Evaluation with visual examination and tissue sampling for infections

Traditionally, ERCP may be of assistance in characterizing strictures by providing tissue sampling; however, the low yield rates of ERCP-based methods for securing diagnosis of malignancy range from 35% to 70%.[42–48] Direct visualization of the biliary ducts using cholangioscopy increases the ability to differentiate and diagnose lesions accurately in comparison with standard imaging or ERCP techniques.[49–53] The combination of POCS and ERCP improved the sensitivity of diagnosing malignant lesions from 58% to 93%. In addition, POCS was useful in evaluating filling defects of uncertain etiology and was able to correctly diagnose malignant and benign lesions with an accuracy of 100%.[52] By evaluating mucosal changes, presence of neovascularization, and patterns of luminal narrowing, it was determined that bile duct tumors demonstrate unique optical characteristics that could allow their differentiation.[50] Another study demonstrated that cholangioscopy could potentially improve the diagnosis of cholangiocarcinoma by allowing the optical recognition of an irregularly dilated and tortuous vessel, the so-called tumor vessel. The presence of tumor vessels had a sensitivity of 61%, but combining the optical observation of tumor vessels with PTCS-guided biopsy resulted in a diagnosis of malignancy in 96% of the patients. The negative predictive value of tumor vessels on a basis of a 1-year follow-up was 100%.[50] Cholangioscopy guides tissue sampling by assessing for tumor vessels, intraductal nodules or masses, infiltrative or ulcerated strictures, and papillary or villous mucosal projections.[7,50,54] Prospective studies have shown that cholangioscopic visualization with and without biopsy has a sensitivity of 89% to 100% and specificity of 87% to 96%.[31,52] PTCS-guided biopsy specimens obtained from bile duct carcinomas showed malignancy in 96%; however, the sensitivity of a single biopsy for the diagnosis of malignancy was only 62%, which demonstrated the requirement for multiple biopsies to obtain a higher diagnostic yield.[14,17,55] In a cohort study sensitivities in detecting cholangiocarcinoma of patients with known cancer was 100% for the polypoid type, 95% for the stenotic type, and 100% when tumor vessel pattern was noted. Tissue sampling obtained from the margins and not from within strictures improved the histologic diagnosis rate of stenotic-type cholangiocarcinoma from 70% to 100%.[56] A retrospective study described the use and yield of POCS, with and without mapping biopsies, to diagnose bile duct carcinoma and to assess the extent of proximal and distal intraepithelial tumor spread (ITS) to guide surgical resection.[53] POCS improved the accuracy in the diagnosis of ITS from 79.5% to 100% and showed a diagnostic accuracy in assessing the extent of ITS of 76.9%, which was increased to 100% by adding mapping biopsies to POCS. Data for the semidisposable cholangioscope system have shown a sensitivity of 53% to 71% and a specificity of 82% to 100% in diagnosing malignancy using SpyGlass-directed biopsy.[39,40] The 2.0-mm working channel of an ultraslim upper endoscope allows the passage of larger biopsy forceps, thus increasing the diagnostic yield during tissue sampling.[32,34] With regard to diagnosing or refuting biliary malignancy and in assessing the extent of the disease, the future belongs to cholangioscopy. Brushings and cholangiographically guided biopsies, whatever additional techniques are applied, simply can never meet the critical precondition for optimal cytologic or histologic diagnosis, which is optimal tissue sampling under direct visual control.[57–60] Future studies specifically designed to compare the diagnostic yield of endoscopic direct cholangioscopy and the semidisposable cholangioscope system with conventional cholangioscopy are pending. In terms of its sensitivity, specificity, accuracy, and positive and negative predictive value, POCS is significantly superior to ERCP in distinguishing between malignant and benign dominant bile duct stenosis in patients with primary sclerosing cholangitis (PSC).[61–63]

Image-enhanced cholangioscopy techniques have been evaluated for use in biliary diseases, including chromocholangioscopy with dye solution, AFI, and NBI in addition to conventional white light illumination. Three studies evaluated the usefulness of POCS or PTCS in biliary tract lesions, using 0.1% methylene blue for better observation.[64–66] The investigators described neoplastic findings showing irregular mucosa with inhomogeneous and intensively dark-blue staining patterns, whereas nonneoplastic findings had a smooth surface mucosa with homogeneous staining.[65] Although chromocholangioscopy has some potential for enhancing visualization of bile duct lesions, the presence of mucus, exudate, bile, or contrast tends to obscure mucosal details and often interferes with the ability to achieve adequate tissue sampling.[67] With autofluorescence cholangioscopy normal mucosa appeared green and neoplastic lesions change from green to dark green or black, owing to differences in the intensity of the autofluorescence. The diagnostic ability of PTCS without and with AFI has shown a sensitivity of 88% and 100%, specificity of 88% and 53%, and accuracy of 88% and 71%.[66] However, the frequency of false-positive results increased with AFI. Nonneoplastic granular mucosa tended to appear slightly dark green and bile was recognized as dark-green fluid. Furthermore, during POCS bile often hindered the field of view because saline irrigation is difficult to achieve through a small working channel. NBI, which is based on the modification of spectral features with an optical color-separation filter narrowing the bandwidth of spectral transmittance, enhances visualization of fine surface mucosal structures and mucosal capillary microvessels compared with white light endoscopy. The pilot studies using NBI in the biliary system only involve a small number of cases.[35,68–71] The delineation of the proximal and distal margins of biliary tract lesions and identification of vessels on the surface of the lesions were evaluated. Significantly better identification of the surface structure and tumor vessels by NBI than with conventional observation was reported (**Fig. 4**A, B).[68] In particular, at the sites of superficial tumor spread, NBI tended to be better than conventional observation at detecting the lesion and delineating the margins.[68,71] Technically challenging is the sufficient removal of abundant bile, mucin, and blood, especially because bile and blood both appear

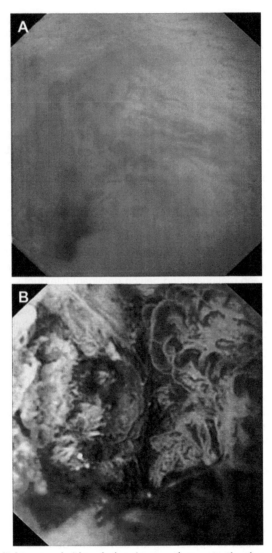

Fig. 4. (*A*) White light peroral video cholangioscopy demonstrating irregular vessels at the distal margin of a cholangiocarcinoma. (*B*) Visualization of the same lesion with NBI showing details of corkscrew-like deformation of tumor vessels.

as dark red in the NBI mode. Another promising imaging modality to improve the preoperative diagnosis of biliary neoplasms is probe-based confocal laser endomicroscopy with confocal miniprobes further miniaturized to enable their use via the instrumentation channel of cholangioscopes.[72–74] In 14 patients the presence of irregular vessels using confocal laser microscopy enabled prediction of neoplasia with an accuracy rate of 86%, sensitivity of 83%, and specificity of 88%; respective accuracy for standard histopathology was 79%.[72] Preliminary clinical experience suggests that these innovative enhanced imaging cholangioscopy techniques may help to distinguish benign from malignant diseases, and highlight certain features such as mucosal structures and mucosal microvessels.

Prospective randomized studies are required to confirm the diagnostic value of these advanced imaging technologies.

In a retrospective series of fiberoptic cholangioscopy and virtual CT cholangioscopy interpreted by radiologists, no significant difference was noted for endoluminal visualization quality.[75] However, CT's detection rate of minute papillary tumors and stones less than 5 mm was significantly lower than cholangioscopy, at 30% to 100% and 25% to 100%, respectively. In another study the sensitivity and specificity of IDUS compared with PTCS in the detection of biliary cancers was 89% versus 93% and 50% versus 100%, respectively.[7] One study demonstrated the highest accuracy in the preoperative evaluation of longitudinal tumor extent of hilar cholangiocarcinomas for PTCS with biopsy (90%), compared with MRC (84%) and IDUS (85%). The accuracy of the combination of IDUS and PTCS with biopsy was 100% in patients with Bismuth type III and IV cancer.[76]

Other diagnostic indications of cholangioscopy include the evaluation of choledochal cysts, hemobilia of unknown etiology, and infectious causes of bile duct pathology, such as cytomegalovirus and fungal infections.[49,77–80]

THERAPEUTIC APPLICATIONS

The therapeutic indications for cholangioscopy include the treatment of difficult biliary stones with or without intraductal lithotripsy,[81–86] palliative therapy for biliary malignancies with PDT,[87] APC[35,88] or Nd-YAG laser ablation,[49] and advancement of guidewires across complex strictures under direct visualization for subsequent balloon dilatation or insertion of stents.[32,36,88]

The main therapeutic applications of cholangioscopy are intraductal EHL and LL for difficult biliary stones. Direct visualization of the stone is required to avoid shock-wave pulses to the bile duct wall, which can lead to bleeding and perforation. The success rate of cholangioscopically guided lithotripsy for complicated choledocholithiasis is high, varying from 80% to 100% (**Fig. 5A, B**).[82–86] In most cases, stone disintegration and complete bile duct clearance can be achieved within a single treatment session. For comparison of extracorporeal shock-wave lithotripsy (ESWL) with POCS and EHL, a nonrandomized study revealed a 79% stone clearance rate in the ESWL group and 74% in the EHL group.[89] Cross-over treatments resulted in successful duct clearance in 94% of patients. A randomized, prospective study demonstrated a higher rate of duct clearance for cholangioscopic-guided LL (97% vs 73%) and a lower number of sessions (1.2 vs 3) than with ESWL.[90] After cross-over therapy 98% of the patients achieved clearance. In comparison with EHL, LL has comparable efficacy but is more expensive and time-consuming.[81,82] However, the laser fiber is significantly thinner than the EHL counterpart and is more appropriate for cholangioscopes with small-caliber accessory channels. Furthermore, LL is especially preferred in cases of intrahepatic stones or stones situated proximal to a bile duct stenosis.[82,84] First results of EHL performed under SpyGlass guidance demonstrated a clearance rate from bile duct stones of 100% after failure of prior conventional ERCP stone extraction.[39] Accordingly, the prospective multicenter study showed an overall success rate of 92%, defined as adequate stone visualization, initiation of stone fragmentation, and removal per SpyGlass-guided EHL or LL.[40] Another prospective trial reported a complete bile duct clearance rate of 77% after a single session of SpyGlass-guided LL in patients in whom conventional endoscopic stone therapy failed.[91] Cases of selective guidewire access and drainage of the gallbladder using the SpyGlass system[92] and SpyGlass-guided EHL through a colonoscope in a patient with Roux-en-Y hepaticojejunostomy[93] have been described. An evaluation of the feasibility of

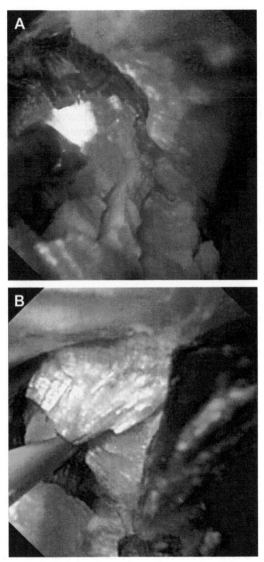

Fig. 5. (A) Video cholangioscopy for laser lithotripsy of an impacted common bile duct stone. The tip of the fiber is on the stone surface, and application of pulsed laser light causes stone fragmentation. (B) Further fragmentation into small pieces.

direct POCS using an ultraslim upper endoscope for EHL or LL by a single endoscopist demonstrated an overall success rate of 89% and an average number of treatment sessions of 1.6.[94]

COMPLICATIONS AND SAFETY

In general, cholangioscopy is safe for both diagnostic and therapeutic purposes, provided that prior sphincterotomy has been performed and that lithotripsy is performed under clear visual control. Complications of cholangioscopy are related to the route of access, hemobilia, and bile leakage due to intraductal lithotripsy, and the introduction of infection into the biliary system, especially in patients with incomplete biliary drainage. POCS with and without intraductal lithotripsy has been associated with cholangitis rates of 0% to 14%,[31,37,39,85,86] hemobilia rates of 0% to 3%,[37,85] and one case of a bile leak.[85] Cholangitis is probably related to intraductal irrigation, which should therefore be minimized especially upstream of ductal obstruction . For intraductal LL, a morbidity of 33% to 40% was noted with PTCS compared with 0% to 20% morbidity with POCS, the latter all being attributable to sphincterotomy.[82,95] In series of PTCS, rates of infectious complications were 8% to 35%,[41,96,97] loss of tract access 1% to 2%,[97,98] and hemobilia 1% to 6%.[41,96,97] The access and maintenance of the percutaneous tract accounts for the higher morbidity rate compared with the peroral cholangioscopy.

SUMMARY

Cholangioscopy is a valuable complementary method in the diagnosis of and therapy for selected biliary disorders. The dissemination of this technology has remained limited to expert centers due to several limitations, such as the challenging techniques, the requirement of extensive experience, and high maintenance costs. Several recent developments offer new options for cholangioscopy. The implementation of video chip technology has improved the image quality of peroral and percutaneous cholangioscopes. The semidisposable SpyGlass system allows enhanced maneuverability and continuous irrigation requiring only a single endoscopist. Especially designed balloon catheters facilitate direct insertion of ultraslim upper endoscopes into the biliary tree, and provide a high image quality and a wider accessory channel for diagnostic and therapeutic applications. Further innovative imaging techniques, such as NBI or AFI and the integration of confocal endomicroscopy, promise improved examination and characterization of the ductal mucosa. Therefore, these new options for cholangioscopic technology justify a wider role in endoscopic practice.

REFERENCES

1. MacEneaney P, Mitchell MT, McDermott R. Update on magnetic resonance cholangiopancreatography. Gastroenterol Clin North Am 2002;31:731–46.
2. Tripathy RP, Batra A, Kaushik S. Magnetic resonance cholangiopancreatography: evaluation in 150 patients. Indian J Gastroenterol 2002;21:105–9.
3. Deveraux CE, Binmoeller KF. Endoscopic retrograde cholangiopancreatography in the next millennium. Gastrointest Endosc Clin N Am 2000;10:117–33.
4. Rösch T, Hofrichter K, Frimberger E, et al. ERCP or EUS for tissue diagnosis of biliary structures? A prospective comparative study. Gastrointest Endosc 2004; 60:390–6.
5. Rösch T, Meining A, Frühmorgen S, et al. A prospective comparison of the diagnostic accuracy of ERCP, MRCP, CT, and EUS in biliary strictures. Gastrointest Endosc 2002;55:870–6.
6. Chak A, Isenberg G, Kobayashi K, et al. Prospective evaluation of an over-the-wire catheter US probe. Gastrointest Endosc 2000;51:202–5.
7. Tamada K, Ueno N, Tomiyama T, et al. Characterization of biliary strictures using intraductal ultrasonography: comparison with percutaneous cholangioscopy biopsy. Gastrointest Endosc 1998;47:341–9.
8. Nakajima M, Akasaka Y, Fukumoto K, et al. Peroral cholangiopancreatoscopy (PCPS) under duodenoscopic guidance. Am J Gastroenterol 1976;66:241–7.
9. Rösch W, Koch H, Demling L. Peroral cholangioscopy. Endoscopy 1976;8:172–5.

10. Takada T, Suzuki S, Nakamura K, et al. Percutaneous transhepatic cholangioscopy as a new approach to the diagnosis of biliary disease. Gastroenterol Endosc 1974;16:106–11.
11. Urakami Y, Seifert E, Butke H. Peroral direct cholangioscopy (PDCS) using routine straight-view endoscope: first report. Endoscopy 1977;9:27–30.
12. Urakami Y. Peroral cholangiopancreatoscopy (PCPS) and peroral direct cholangioscopy (PDCS). Endoscopy 1980;12:30–7.
13. Bogardus ST, Hanan I, Ruchim M, et al. "Mother-baby" biliary endoscopy: the University of Chicago experience. Am J Gastroenterol 1996;91:105–10.
14. Kozarek R, Kodama T, Tatsumi Y. Direct cholangioscopy and pancreatoscopy. Gastrointest Endosc Clin N Am 2003;13:593–607.
15. Allescher HD, Neuhaus H, Hagenmueller F, et al. Effect of N-butylscopolamine on sphincter of Oddi motility in patients during routine ERCP—a manometric study. Endoscopy 1990;22:160–3.
16. Rey JF, Greff M, Picazo J. Glucagon-(1-21)-peptide. Study of its action on sphincter of Oddi function by endoscopic manometry. Dig Dis Sci 1986;31:355–60.
17. Kozarek R. Direct cholangioscopy and pancreatoscopy at time of endoscopic retrograde cholangiopancreatography. Am J Gastroenterol 1988;83:55–7.
18. Foerster EC, Schneider MU, Stommer P, et al. Miniscopes in gastroenterological endoscopy—inspection of the gallbladder and the biliary and pancreatic duct systems in autopsy specimens. Endoscopy 1988;20:316–20.
19. Bourke MJ, Haber GB. Transpapillary choledochoscopy. Gastrointest Endosc Clin N Am 1996;6:235–52.
20. Neuhaus H, Schumacher B. Miniscopes. Baillieres Best Pract Res Clin Gastroenterol 1999;13:33–48.
21. Soda K, Yamanaka T, Yoshida Y, et al. A newly developed fine-caliber endoscope for peroral cholangiopancreatoscopy. Endoscopy 1994;26:671–5.
22. Soda K, Shitou K, Yoshida Y, et al. Peroral cholangioscopy using a new fine-caliber flexible scope for detailed examination without papillotomy. Gastrointest Endosc 1996;43:233–8.
23. Sander R, Poesl H. Initial experience with a new babyscope for endoscopic retrograde cholangiopancreatoscopy. Gastrointest Endosc 1996;44:191–4.
24. American Society for Gastrointestinal Endoscopy (ASGE). Duodenoscope-assisted Cholangiopancreatoscopy. Gastrointest Endosc 1999;50:943–5.
25. Shim CS, Neuhaus H, Tamada K. Direct cholangioscopy. Endoscopy 2003;35:752–8.
26. Meenan J, Schoeman M, Rauws E, et al. A video baby cholangioscope. Gastrointest Endosc 1995;42:584–5.
27. Kodama T, Koshitani T, Sato H, et al. Electronic pancreatoscopy for the diagnosis of pancreatic diseases. Am J Gastroenterol 2002;97:617–22.
28. Kodama T, Imamura Y, Sato H, et al. Feasibility study using a new small electronic pancreatoscope: description of findings in chronic pancreatitis. Endoscopy 2003;35:305–10.
29. Kodama T, Tatsumi Y, Sato H, et al. Initial experience with a new peroral electronic pancreatoscope with an accessory channel. Gastrointest Endosc 2004;59:895–900.
30. Nguyen NQ, Binmoeller KF, Shah JN. Cholangioscopy and pancreatoscopy. Gastrointest Endosc 2009;70:1200–10.
31. Shah RJ, Langer DA, Antillon MR, et al. Cholangioscopy and cholangioscopic forceps biopsy in patients with indeterminate pancreaticobiliary pathology. Clin Gastroenterol Hepatol 2006;4:219–25.

32. Larghi A, Waxman I. Endoscopic direct cholangioscopy by using an ultra-slim upper endoscope: a feasibility study. Gastrointest Endosc 2006;63:853–7.
33. Choi HJ, Moon JH, Ko BM, et al. Overtube-balloon-assisted direct peroral cholangioscopy by using an ultra-slim upper endoscope. Gastrointest Endosc 2009;69:935–40.
34. Moon JH, Ko BM, Choi HJ, et al. Intraductal balloon-guided direct peroral cholangioscopy with an ultraslim upper endoscope. Gastrointest Endosc 2009;70:297–302.
35. Brauer BC, Fukami N, Chen YK. Direct cholangioscopy with narrow-band imaging, chromoscopy and argon plasma coagulation of intraductal papillary mucinous neoplasm of the bile duct. Gastrointest Endosc 2008;67:574–6.
36. Waxman I, Chennant J, Konda V. Peroral direct cholangioscopic-guided selective intrahepatic duct stent placement with an ultraslim endoscope. Gastrointest Endosc 2010;71:875–8.
37. Farrell JJ, Bounds BC, Al-Shalabi S, et al. Single-operator duodenoscope-assisted cholangioscopy is an effective alternative in the management of choledocholithiasis not removed by conventional methods, including mechanical lithotripsy. Endoscopy 2005;37:542–7.
38. Chen YK. Preclinical characterization of the SpyGlass peroral cholangiopancreatoscopy system for direct access, visualization, and biopsy. Gastrointest Endosc 2007;65:303–11.
39. Chen YK, Pleskow DK. SpyGlass single-operator peroral cholangiopancreatoscopy system for the diagnosis and therapy of bile-duct disorders: a clinical feasibility study. Gastrointest Endosc 2007;65:832–41.
40. Neuhaus H, Parsi MA, Chen YK, et al. Peroral cholangioscopy for biliary strictures and bile duct stones—an international registry using SpyGlass. Abstract UEGW 2009.
41. Simon T, Fink AS, Zuckerman AM, et al. Experience with percutaneous transhepatic cholangioscopy in the management of biliary tract disease. Surg Endosc 1999;13:1199–202.
42. Glasbrenner B, Ardan M, Boeck W, et al. Prospective evaluation of brush cytology of biliary strictures during endoscopic retrograde cholangiopancreatography. Endoscopy 1999;31:712–7.
43. Jailwala J, Fogel EL, Sherman S, et al. Triple-tissue sampling at ERCP in malignant biliary obstruction. Gastrointest Endosc 2000;51:383–90.
44. Ponchon T, Gagnon P, Berger F, et al. Value of endobiliary brush cytology and biopsies for the diagnosis of malignant bile duct stenosis: results of a prospective study. Gastrointest Endosc 1995;42:565–72.
45. Pugliese V, Conio M, Nicolo G, et al. Endoscopic retrograde forceps biopsy and brush cytology of biliary strictures: a prospective study. Gastrointest Endosc 1995;42:520–6.
46. Sugiyama M, Atomi Y, Wada N, et al. Endoscopic transpapillary bile duct biopsy without sphincterotomy for diagnosing biliary strictures: a prospective comparative study with bile and brush cytology. Am J Gastroenterol 1996;91:465–7.
47. Schoefl R, Haefner M, Wrba F, et al. Forceps biopsy and brush cytology during endoscopic retrograde cholangiopancreatography for the diagnosis of biliary stenoses. Scand J Gastroenterol 1997;32:363–8.
48. Stewart CJ, Mills PR, Carter R, et al. Brush cytology in the assessment of pancreato-biliary strictures: a review of 460 cases. J Clin Pathol 2001;54:449–55.
49. Siddique I, Galati J, Ankoma-Sey V, et al. The role of choledochoscopy in the diagnosis and management of biliary tract diseases. Gastrointest Endosc 1999;50:67–73.

50. Seo DW, Lee SK, Yoo KS, et al. Cholangioscopic findings in bile duct tumors. Gastrointest Endosc 2000;52:630–4.
51. Kim HJ, Kim MH, Lee SK, et al. Tumor vessel: a valuable cholangioscopic clue of malignant biliary stricture. Gastrointest Endosc 2000;52:635–8.
52. Fukuda Y, Tsuyuguchi T, Sakai Y, et al. Diagnostic utility of peroral cholangioscopy for various bile-duct lesions. Gastrointest Endosc 2005;62:374–82.
53. Kawakami H, Kuwatani M, Etoh K, et al. Endoscopic retrograde cholangiography versus peroral cholangioscopy to evaluate intraepithelial tumor spread in biliary cancer. Endoscopy 2009;11:959–64.
54. Somogyi L, Dimashkieh H, Weber FL, et al. Biliary intraductal papillary mucinous tumor: diagnosis and localization by endoscopic retrograde cholangioscopy. Gastrointest Endosc 2003;57:620–2.
55. Sato M, Inoue H, Ogawa S, et al. Limitations of percutaneous transhepatic cholangioscopy for the diagnosis of the intramural extension of bile duct carcinoma. Endoscopy 1998;30:281–8.
56. Tamada K, Kurihara K, Tomiyama T, et al. How many biopsies should be performed during percutaneous transhepatic cholangioscopy to diagnose biliary tract cancer? Gastrointest Endosc 1999;50:653–8.
57. Bruno MJ. Diagnosing and staging bile duct cancer: cholangiographically guided biopsies or cholangioscopy? Endoscopy 2009;41:991–2.
58. Iqbal S, Stevens PD. Cholangiopancreatoscopy for targeted biopsies of bile and pancreatic ducts. Gastrointest Endosc Clin N Am 2009;19:567–77.
59. Nimura Y. Staging of cholangiocarcinoma by cholangioscopy. HPB (Oxford) 2008;10:113–5.
60. Weber A, Schmid RM, Prinz C. Diagnostic approaches for cholangiocarcinoma. World J Gastroenterol 2008;14:4131–6.
61. Awadallah NS, Chen YK, Piraka C, et al. Is there a role for cholangioscopy in patients with primary sclerosing cholangitis? Am J Gastroenterol 2006;101: 284–91.
62. Tischendorf JJ, Kruger M, Trautwein C, et al. Cholangioscopic characterization of dominant bile duct stenoses in patients with primary sclerosing cholangitis. Endoscopy 2006;38:665–9.
63. Petersen BT. Cholangioscopy for special applications: primary sclerosing cholangitis, liver transplant, and selective duct access. Gastrointest Endosc Clin N Am 2009;19:579–86.
64. Maetani I, Ogawa S, Sato M, et al. Lack of methylene blue staining in superficial epithelia as a possible marker for superficial lateral spread of bile duct cancer. Diagn Ther Endosc 1996;3:29–34.
65. Hoffmann A, Kiesslich R, Bittinger F, et al. Methylene blue-aided cholangioscopy in patients with biliary strictures: feasibility and outcome analysis. Endoscopy 2008;40:563–71.
66. Itoi T, Shinohara S, Takeda K, et al. Improvement of choledochoscopy-chromoendoscopy, autofluorescense imaging, or narrow-band imaging. Dig Endosc 2007; 19:S95–102.
67. Itoi T, Neuhaus H, Chen YK. Diagnostic value of image-enhanced video cholangiopancreatoscopy. Gastrointest Endosc Clin N Am 2009;19:557–66.
68. Itoi T, Sofuni A, Itokawa F, et al. Peroral cholangioscopic diagnosis of biliary tract diseases using narrow-band imaging. Gastrointest Endosc 2007;66:730–6.
69. Itoi T, Sofuni A, Itokawa F, et al. Evaluation of peroral cholangioscopy using narrow-band imaging for diagnosis of intraductal papillary neoplasm of the bile duct. Dig Endosc 2009;21:S103–7.

70. Igarashi Y, Okano N, Ito K, et al. Effectiveness of peroral cholangioscopy and narrow band imaging for endoscopically diagnosing the bile duct cancer. Dig Endosc 2009;21:S101–2.
71. Lu XL, Itoi T, Kubota K. Cholangioscopy using narrow band imaging and transpapillary radiotherapy for mucin-producing bile duct tumor. Clin Gastroenterol Hepatol 2009;7:e34–5.
72. Meining A, Frimberger E, Becker V, et al. Detection of cholangiocarcinoma in vivo using miniprobe-based confocal fluorescence microscopy. Clin Gastroenterol Hepatol 2008;6:1057–60.
73. Wallace MB, Fockens P. Probe-based confocal laser endomicroscopy. Gastroenterology 2009;136:1509–13.
74. Meining A. Confocal endomicroscopy. Gastrointest Endosc Clin N Am 2009;19: 629–35.
75. Koito K, Namieno T, Hirokawa N, et al. Virtual CT cholangioscopy: comparison with fiberoptic cholangioscopy. Endoscopy 2001;33:676–81.
76. Kim HM, Park JY, Kim KS, et al. Intraductal ultrasonography combined with percutaneous transhepatic cholangioscopy for the preoperative evaluation of longitudinal tumor extent in hilar cholangiocarcinoma. J Gastroenterol Hepatol 2010;25:286–92.
77. Kolodziejski TR, Safadi BY, Nakanuma Y, et al. Bile duct cysts in a patient with autosomal dominant polycystic kidney disease. Gastrointest Endosc 2004;59: 140–2.
78. Scotiniotis IA, Kochmann ML. Intramural cyst of the bile duct demonstrated by cholangioscopy and intraductal US. Gastrointest Endosc 2001;54:260–2.
79. Kubota H, Kageoka M, Iwasaki H, et al. A patient with undifferentiated carcinoma of gallbladder presenting with hemobilia. J Gastroenterol 2000;35:63–8.
80. Prasad GA, Abraham SC, Baron TH, et al. Hemobilia caused by cytomegalovirus cholangiopathy. Am J Gastroenterol 2005;100:2592–5.
81. Neuhaus H. Cholangioscopy. Endoscopy 1994;26:120–5.
82. Neuhaus H, Hoffmann W, Zillinger C, et al. Laser lithotripsy of difficult bile duct stones under direct visual control. Gut 1993;34:415–21.
83. Binmoeller KF, Bruckner M, Thonke F, et al. Treatment of difficult bile duct stones using mechanical, electrohydraulic and extracorporeal shock wave lithotripsy. Endoscopy 1993;25:201–6.
84. Jakobs R, Pereira-Lima JC, Schuch AW, et al. Endoscopic laser lithotripsy for complicated bile duct stones: is cholangioscopic guidance necessary? Arq Gastroenterol 2007;44:137–40.
85. Arya N, Nelles SE, Haber GB, et al. Electrohydraulic lithotripsy in 111 patients: a safe and effective therapy for difficult bile duct stones. Am J Gastroenterol 2004;99:2330–4.
86. Piraka C, Shah RJ, Awadallah NS, et al. Transpapillary cholangioscopy directed lithotripsy in patients with difficult bile duct stones. Clin Gastroenterol Hepatol 2007;5:1333–8.
87. Shim CS, Cheon YK, Cha SW, et al. Prospective study of the effectiveness of percutaneous transhepatic photodynamic therapy for advanced bile duct cancer and the role of intraductal ultrasonography in response assessment. Endoscopy 2005;37:425–33.
88. Park do H, Park BW, Lee HS, et al. Peroral direct cholangioscopic argon plasma coagulation by using an ultraslim upper endoscope for recurrent hepatoma with intraductal nodular tumor growth. Gastrointest Endosc 2007;66: 201–3.

89. Adamek HE, Maier M, Jakobs R, et al. Management of retained bile duct stones: a prospective open trial comparing extracorporeal and intracorporeal lithotripsy. Gastrointest Endosc 1996;44:40–7.

90. Neuhaus H, Zillinger C, Born P, et al. Randomized, study of intracorporeal laser lithotripsy versus extracorporeal shock-wave lithotripsy for difficult bile duct stones. Gastrointest Endosc 1998;47:327–34.

91. Seelhoff A, Schumacher B, Neuhaus H, et al. Prospective study of SpyGlass guided laser lithotripsy of bile duct stones after failure of conventional endoscopic techniques. Abstract DDW 2009.

92. Barkay O, Bucksot L, Sherman S. Endoscopic transpapillary gallbladder drainage with the SpyGlass cholangiopancreatoscopy system. Gastrointest Endosc 2009;70:1039–40.

93. Baron TH, Saleem A. Intraductal electrohydraulic lithotripsy by using SpyGlass cholangioscopy through a colonoscope in a patient with Roux-en-Y hepaticojejunostomy. Gastrointest Endosc 2010;71:650–1.

94. Moon JH, Ko BM, Choi HJ, et al. Direct peroral cholangioscopy using an ultra-slim upper endoscope for the treatment of retained bile duct stones. Am J Gastroenterol 2009;104:2729–33.

95. Ponchon T, Gagnon P, Valette PJ, et al. Pulsed dye laser lithotripsy of bile duct stones. Gastroenterology 1991;100:1730–6.

96. Lee SK, Seo DW, Myung SJ, et al. Percutaneous transhepatic cholangioscopic treatment for hepatolithiasis: an evaluation of long-term results and risk factors for recurrence. Gastrointest Endosc 2001;53:318–21.

97. Yeh YH, Huang MH, Yang JC, et al. Percutaneous transhepatic cholangioscopy and lithotripsy in the treatment of intrahepatic stones: a study with 5-year-follow-up. Gastrointest Endosc 1995;42:13–8.

98. Oh HC, Lee SK, Lee TY, et al. Analysis of percutaneous transhepatic cholangioscopy-related complications and the risk factors for those complications. Endoscopy 2007;39:731–6.

Contrast-Enhanced and 3-Dimensional Endoscopic Ultrasonography

Marc Giovannini, MD, PH

KEYWORDS

- Microbubbles • Enhancement of vascularization
- Power Doppler • Harmonic imaging • 3D EUS
- Pancreatic mass • Lymph nodes

Recent progress of the data processing applied to ultrasonographic (US) examination has made it possible to develop new software. The US workstation of the last generation thus incorporated in their center a computer allowing a precise treatment of the US image. This advancement has made it possible to work out new images such as 3-dimensional (3D) US, contrast harmonic US associated with the intravenous (IV) injection of contrast agents, and more recently, elastography. These techniques, quite elaborate in percutaneous US at present, are to be adapted and evaluated with endoscopic US (EUS).

The contribution of the contrast agents of US to pancreatic EUS and then 3D EUS are successively approached in this article.

CONTRAST-ENHANCED EUS

Among several technologies, EUS has been widely used to diagnose pancreatic, lymph node, and gastrointestinal (GI) tumors because EUS is superior to any other modality with respect to spatial resolution. However, EUS has limitations in evaluating vascularity by contrast US when the color Doppler or power Doppler mode is used. Contrast-enhanced power Doppler US is accompanied by artifacts, for example, blooming, so that the width of a blood vessel visualized by the power Doppler mode is magnified and wider than that visualized by fundamental B-mode imaging. Contrast harmonic imaging by IV infusion of Levovist (SHU508 A), an air-filled microbubble with an outer shell composed of 99.9% galactose and 0.1% palmitic acid, has allowed the observation of the vasculature of the abdominal organs on transabdominal US. If the US equipment receives harmonic components that are integer multiples of the fundamental frequency, then the harmonic content derived from microbubbles is higher than that from tissues. Contrast harmonic imaging detects signals from microbubbles and filters the signals that originate from tissue by selectively detecting the

Paoli-Calmettes Institute, 232 Boulevard Sainte Marguerite, 13273 Marseille Cedex 9, France
E-mail address: uemco@marseille.fnclcc.fr

Gastroenterol Clin N Am 39 (2010) 845–858
doi:10.1016/j.gtc.2010.08.027
0889-8553/10/$ – see front matter © 2010 Published by Elsevier Inc.

gastro.theclinics.com

harmonic components. This technology can detect signals from microbubbles in vessels with a very slow flow without Doppler-related artifacts and is used to characterize tumor vascularity in liver, pancreas, gallbladder, and GI tract during transabdominal US. Until recently, there was no contrast harmonic imaging available for EUS examination because the transducer for current echoendoscopes is of a limited frequency bandwidth and is too small to produce enough acoustic power for contrast harmonic imaging when using Levovist. Second-generation US contrast agents (UCAs), for example, SonoVue, produce harmonic signals at lower acoustic powers and, therefore, are suitable for EUS at low acoustic powers.

General Considerations

UCAs, in conjunction with contrast-specific imaging, are increasingly accepted in clinical use for diagnostic imaging and postinterventional workup in several organs. To those not closely involved in the field, the rapid advances in technology and techniques can be difficult to follow. In March 2003, at the European Federation of Societies for Ultrasound (EUROSON) Congress in Copenhagen, it was agreed that it would be useful to produce a document providing a description of essential technical requirements, proposed investigator qualifications, suggested study procedures and steps, guidance on image interpretation, and recommended and established clinical indications and safety considerations.[1]

The development of UCAs, which perform as blood pool tracers, has overcome the limitations of conventional B-mode and color Doppler or power Doppler US and enable the display of parenchymal microvasculature.[2] Depending on the contrast agent and the mode of US, the dynamic lesion enhancement pattern is visualized during intermittent or continuous imaging. Enhancement patterns are described during subsequent vascular phases (eg, arterial, portal venous, and late phases for liver lesions), similar to contrast-enhanced computed tomography (CECT) and/or contrast-enhanced magnetic resonance imaging (CEMRI). Contrast-enhanced US (CEUS) and CECT or CEMRI are not equivalent because UCAs have different pharmacokinetics and are confined to the intravascular space, whereas most of the currently approved contrast agents for CT and MRI are rapidly cleared from the blood pool into the extracellular space.

An inherent advantage of CEUS is the possibility to assess the contrast enhancement patterns in real time with a substantially higher temporal resolution than other imaging modalities and without the need to predefine time points of scans or perform bolus tracking. Furthermore, administration of UCAs can be repeated because of the excellent patient tolerance to them.

In addition to IV use, intracavity applications of the UCAs, such as intravesical administration, can be performed.

Studies on Ultrasound Contrast Agents are subject to the same limitations as other types of US studies. As a general rule, if the baseline result of US is very suboptimal, CEUS may be disappointing.

Commercially Available UCAs in Europe

At present, 4 transpulmonary UCAs are approved and marketed within European Countries:

1. Levovist (air filled, with galactose and palmitic acid as a surfactant; introduced in 1996). Main indications include vesicoureteric reflux and cardiac, abdominal, and transcranial applications.

2. Optison (octafluoropropane (perflutren) with an albumin shell; introduced in 1998). Sole indication to date is in cardiac applications.
3. SonoVue (sulfur hexafluoride with a phospholipid shell; introduced in 2001). Approved indications are cardiac (endocardial border delineation), macrovascular (cerebral and peripheral arteries, portal vein), and microvascular (characterization of focal lesions in liver, pancreas, and breast).
4. Luminity (octafluoropropane perflutren with a lipid shell; introduced in 2006). Sole indication to date is in cardiac applications.

There are other UCAs that are approved outside Europe or under investigation.

The UCAs that are used at present in diagnostic US are characterized by a micro-bubble structure consisting of gas bubbles stabilized by a shell. UCAs act as blood pool agents. They strongly increase the US backscatter and therefore are useful in the enhancement of echogenicity for the assessment of blood flow. Although conventional US can detect high concentrations of microbubbles, in practice, their assessment usually requires contrast-specific imaging modes.

Contrast-specific US modes are generally based on the cancellation and/or separation of linear US signals from tissue and use of the nonlinear response from microbubbles.

Nonlinear response from microbubbles is based on 2 different mechanisms:

1. Nonlinear response from microbubble oscillations at low acoustic pressure, chosen to minimize disruption of the microbubbles.
2. High-energy, broadband, nonlinear response arising from microbubble disruption. Nonlinear harmonic US signals may also arise in tissues because of a distortion of the sound wave during its propagation through the tissue. The extent of this harmonic response from the tissue at a given frequency increases with the acoustic pressure, which is proportional to the mechanical index (MI).

Low-solubility gas UCAs (eg, SonoVue, Optison, Luminity) are characterized by the combination of improved stability with favorable resonance behavior at low acoustic pressure. This combination allows minimally disruptive contrast-specific imaging at low MI and enables effective investigations over several minutes with the visualization of the dynamic enhancement pattern in real time. Low-MI techniques, furthermore, lead to effective tissue-signal suppression because the nonlinear response from the tissue is minimal when low acoustic pressures are used. US imaging with air-filled microbubbles (eg, Levovist) at high pressure depends on microbubble disruption, which is a significant limitation for real-time imaging.

Pancreatic EUS and UCAs

Diagnosis between adenocarcinomas and nodular chronic pancreatitis is problematic. All methods of diagnosis are limited. Histology is the standard diagnosis, but even biopsy can be difficult because cancers can produce a marked fibrotic reaction or necrosis and give false results. When there is a stenosis of the main pancreatic duct, the sensitivity and specificity of endoscopic retrograde cholangiopancreatography (ERCP) are 85% and 66%, respectively.[3] Magnetic resonance cholangiopancreatography (MRCP) has a similar sensitivity and specificity as that of ERCP for detecting pancreatic cancer or chronic pancreatitis.

Nevertheless, sensitivity is yet to be perfectible, and MRCP gives a correct differentiation between malignant and benign lesions in 58% of the cases.[4,5] MRCP remains as an expensive procedure, is time-consuming, and is available only in a few centers.

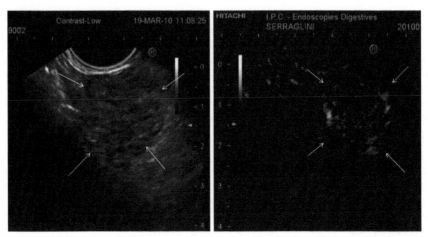

Fig. 1. EUS aspects of endocrine tumor of the pancreas (*arrows*). Enhancement of the micro-vascularization after SonoVue injection.

There are few studies about contrast-enhanced EUS (CE-EUS). Bhutani and colleagues[6] evaluated the utility of Levovist and concluded that it could potentially improve the accuracy of EUS in the diagnosis of malignant vascular invasion, detection of occult pancreatic neoplasms, and diagnosis of vascular thrombosis. Subsequently, Hirooka and colleagues[7] studied the presence or absence of enhancement of different lesions with Albunex in 37 patients. An enhancement of the lesion was observed in 100% of the patients with islet cell tumor (**Fig. 1**), 80% with intraductal papillary mucinous tumor (IPMT), and 75% with chronic pancreatitis and no enhancement effect was observed in the patients with carcinoma (**Fig. 2**). All patients underwent angiography, and comparison between images of CE-EUS and angiography showed similar results, except for 3 patients (2 with IPMT and 1 with chronic pancreatitis) in whom angiograms showed hypovascularity, but enhancement effect was

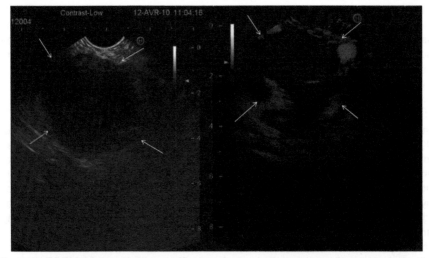

Fig. 2. No enhancement of the mass vascularization with peripheral hypervascularization after contrast injection. CE-EUS image of pancreatic adenocarcinoma (*arrows*).

observed on EUS images. Becker and colleagues[8] evaluated 23 patients with another contrast agent (FS 069 Optison) and evaluated CE-EUS as a method of differentiating inflammation and carcinoma based on perfusion characteristics. Markedly hyperperfused lesions were considered as inflammatory pseudotumors, whereas lesions that were hypoperfused than the surrounding tissue were considered as carcinomas. For the differentiation of pancreatic carcinoma and inflammatory changes the sensitivity was 94%, specificity 100%, positive predictive value (PPV) 100%, and negative predictive value (NPV) 88%. These results are similar to that obtained by Giovannini[9] (sensitivity 90.9%, specificity 88.8%, PPV 88.2%, and NPV 91.4%). Giovannini[9] also studied hyperechoic lesions (supposed not to be a pancreatic adenocarcinoma), and the sensitivity was 88.8%, specificity 90.9%, PPV 91.4%, and NPV 88.2%. In future, CE-EUS could provide a direct and reliable result (malignant or not) without the need to wait several days for histologic findings. Perhaps, CE-EUS could also save time and money in limiting the use of expensive EUS needles. CE-EUS could be an interesting complement to EUS fine-needle aspiration (EUS-FNA) concerning diagnostic accuracy. The sensitivity and diagnostic accuracy of EUS-FNA are 75% to 92% and 79% to 92%, respectively.[8,10–16] First reason, EUS-FNA is not realizable in 6% to 9% of cases owing to vessel interpositions, duodenal stenosis, and tumor hardness, particularly in chronic pancreatitis. Sensitivity of EUS-FNA is limited by uninterpretable material (bleeding or noncellular samples), ranging from 9% to 19% of cases. Totally, the lack of sensitivity of EUS-FNA ranges from 8% to 25% of cases.[8] In the study by Hocke and colleagues,[3] sensitivity and diagnostic accuracy of this technique were comparable to cytopathologic results guided by EUS (sensitivity 90.9%, specificity 88.8%, PPV 88.2%, and NPV 91.4%). From a more general point of view, 97% of hypoechoic lesions were malignant tumors (30 adenocarcinomas, 1 endocrine tumor, 1 pancreatic lymphoma, and 1 pancreatic metastasis from colonic cancer). Therefore, CE-EUS could be a reliable and complementary tool for EUS-FNA in the detection and classification of pancreatic lesions when performing EUS-FNA is impossible or biopsy results are uninterpretable. CE-EUS could improve accuracy and allows to propose an appropriate treatment (eg, surgery, follow-up, chemotherapy).

CE-EUS could differentiate a malign tumor from a pseudotumoral nodule (**Fig. 3**). Chronic pancreatitis is also a limiting factor for diagnosis of pancreatic masses. Several studies have attempted to establish imaging criteria for EUS (without tissue sampling) for differentiating benign inflammatory pseudotumors and tumors. Despite the high resolution of EUS, it does not provide reliable differentiation of benign and malignant lesions of the pancreas.[17] Fritscher-Ravens and colleagues[18] found that the sensitivity of EUS-FNA in patients with a focal pancreatic lesion without chronic pancreatitis was 89%, whereas it was only 54% in patients with chronic pancreatitis. Nevertheless, diagnosis of EUS-FNA influenced clinical management in nearly half of the patients.[19] CE-EUS could also play an important part in the case of lesions occurring within chronic pancreatitis. Indeed, in the study of Hocke and colleagues,[3] adenocarcinoma that developed on chronic pancreatitis was nonenhanced after contrast injection. Conversely, pseudotumoral nodule (benign masses) (91%) in chronic pancreatitis was hypervascularized after SonoVue injection. These results are different and better than studies with CE-EUS. In the study by Takeda and colleagues,[20] 100% of the masses of pseudotumoral pancreatitis had an isoenhanced pattern and it was difficult to differentiate adenocarcinomas from inflammatory pancreatic mass (50% were not well classified).

CE-EUS could be useful in the case of negative results after EUS-FNA. In early studies, NPV of EUS-FNA was around 75%,[13,14] but most recent studies found NPV

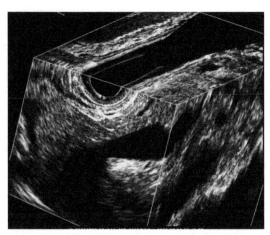

Fig. 3. Normal 3D reconstruction of normal pancreas using an electronic radial probe (PEN-TAX-EG 3670UKR, Pentax Company, Hambourg Germany).

to be between 26% and 44%.[8,10–15] In the study by Oshikawa and colleagues,[21] the rate of patients with negative results of the first biopsy but with malignant tumor diagnosed a second time with a new puncture or surgery, was 47%.

To conclude, the NPV of pancreatic EUS-FNA is 30% to 33%. Theoretically, a new puncture is mandatory to be sure that it is normal tissue. CE-EUS could avoid this second procedure. With regard to false-negative results with SonoVue, 3 adenocarcinomas were found that presented hyperechoic aspect (contrast-enhancement pattern), 2 of which were poorly differentiated adenocarcinomas and the third was associated with IMPT. This finding suggests that poorly differentiated adenocarcinoma could have different vascularity than well-differentiated adenocarcinoma. These results were similar to studies with CE-EUS.[22,23] Differences in histologic findings, such as histologic differentiation grade, amount of fibrosis, and obliteration of blood vessels in the tumor, may be associated with differences in enhancement behavior.

Concerning CE-EUS and endocrine tumors, there is only 1 case report using Levovist that seems to be a useful diagnostic method for precise localization of small insulinoma.[24] In the study by Hocke and colleagues,[3] 87.5% (7 of 8) of endocrine tumors had a strong contrast-enhancement pattern, indicating hypervascular lesions. These results were similar to studies with CE-EUS.[18,22,23,25] These vascular images differed from those of almost all pancreatic ductal carcinomas. Thus, differentiation of enhancement pattern on CE-EUS between pancreatic adenocarcinomas and endocrine tumors is useful in the diagnosis of these lesions. In addition, standard EUS is already known to have a great value for localizing endocrine pancreatic tumors because of its excellent capacity to visualize small lesions and tumor vascularization at the same time.[26,27] Therefore, CE-EUS could increase sensitivity of diagnosis of pancreatic tumors.

Regarding IPMT, in the study by Hocke and colleagues,[3] the only benign tumor was hyperechoic, whereas in malignant IPMT, one was hypoechoic and another was hyperechoic. In the studies on CE-EUS, malignancy could be associated with contrast enhancement. In the study by Sofuni and colleagues,[22] in all 4 patients with IPMT, hypervascularity of the nodules inside the tumors was observed. In the study by Nagase and colleagues,[23] 2 of the 5 IPMTs had solid components within the tumors, and they were positive for enhancement effects. All 5 patients with IPMT underwent surgical resection, and pathologic examination revealed malignancy in the 2 lesions with solid components and positive enhancement. Itoh and colleagues[28] observed that when patients with carcinoma were compared with those with adenoma, the postenhancement intensity was significantly higher in the carcinoma group. CE-EUS could be useful for the differential diagnosis of benign and malignant IPMT. However, the small number of patients with IMPT in each study did not allow conclusions to be made.

Metastatic lesions of the pancreas are rare, between 5% and 10%,[29] but they are an important cause of focal pancreatic lesions. There is only one description of one case of kidney metastasis analyzed by CE-EUS.[30] The study by Giovannini[9] is the first in the literature that describes the enhancement pattern of pancreatic metastasis in CE-EUS. All metastasis except 1 (4 of 5; 80%) showed an echoenhancement pattern, probably proving their hypervascularization. The only nonenhanced pancreatic metastasis was from colonic cancer. CE-EUS could contribute to the differential diagnosis between a primary pancreatic carcinoma and pancreatic metastasis and therefore can have a decisive influence on the selection of appropriate therapeutic strategies (eg, chemotherapy rather than surgery). However, histology remains the standard diagnosis in the differential diagnosis of pancreatic tumors.

CE-EUS in Discrimination Between Benign and Malignant Mediastinal and Abdominal Lymph Nodes

Presence of enlarged mediastinal or abdominal lymph nodes without causing disease is nowadays a clinical issue because of the rapid development of imaging with an increasingly higher resolution of intrathoracic or intra-abdominal structures. At present, CT scanners reliably recognize lymph nodes of 5 to 10 mm in size but do not distinguish between malignant and benign lymph nodes in most cases. EUS has an even higher local resolution, but again, given a distinct visible lymph node, the investigator is frequently not able to assign this node to a malignancy, whether or not a malignant tumor is already known. There are several US features such as size, round shape, hypoechoic appearance, missing hilus sign, and clear borders, which cumulatively make a malignant lymph node most likely. But on the one hand, the specificity of these signs is still less than 90%, and on the other hand, most malignant lymph nodes do not exhibit all these signs simultaneously. EUS-FNA represents the current gold standard and has replaced more invasive procedures such as mediastinoscopy, at least for those groups of lymph nodes that are in reach of the EUS. In case of trained investigators, EUS-FNA reaches a sensitivity, specificity, and diagnostic accuracy of more than 90%. Hocke and colleagues[31] had investigated a total of 122 patients with enlarged mediastinal and/or paraaortic lymph nodes diagnosed by CT. EUS-FNA was performed, and cytologic specimens were diagnosed as representing a malignant or benign process in case of Papanicolaou IV and V or Papanicolaou I and II, respectively. Based on cytologic results, the investigated lymph nodes were classified as neoplastic (n = 48) or nonneoplastic. Using the B-mode criteria, the preliminary diagnosis was confirmed in 64 of 74 benign lymph nodes (specificity 86%). Regarding malignant lymph nodes, 33 of 48 were confirmed (sensitivity 68%). Using the advanced CE-EUS criteria, the diagnosis was confirmed in 68 of 74 benign lymph nodes (specificity 91%). However, in case of malignant lymph nodes, the number of correct diagnoses reduced to 29 of 48 lymph nodes (sensitivity 60%). The CE-EUS criteria to identify benign lymph nodes and node enlargement in malignant lymphoma do not differ. If those 10 patients with malignant lymphoma are excluded, the sensitivity of the CE-EUS for malignant lymph nodes increases to 73%. CE-EUS improves the specificity in diagnosing benign lymph nodes as compared with B-mode EUS. It does not improve the correct identification of malignant lymph nodes and cannot replace EUS-FNA.[32]

Summary

CE-EUS could provide a contribution to the differential diagnosis of a primary pancreatic carcinoma, chronic pancreatitis, and a pancreatic metastasis; therefore, CE-EUS can have a decisive influence on the selection of appropriate therapeutic strategies (eg, follow-up, chemotherapy, or surgery). However, histology remains the standard method in the differential diagnosis of pancreatic tumors. Regarding lymph nodes, CE-EUS cannot replace EUS-FNA.

THREE-DIMENSIONAL EUS

Recent development of the probes of electronic echoendoscopy connected to the US machine of last generation, such as Hitachi Company, Tokyo, Japan 7500, 900, or Prerius, with a built-in 3D software makes it possible to obtain EUS images very easily at present. The acquisition of the images is very fast, approximately 30 seconds; the 2-dimensional (2D) images are rebuilt in 6 plans different by the computer from the US machine. The images are returned in a 3D volume of cubic form, thus making it possible to build transverse and longitudinal cuts of the 6 faces of the cube (see **Fig. 3**).

The swift acquisition of the images makes it possible to eliminate all the artifacts, in particular on the level of the mediastinum (**Fig. 4**), those induced by the cardiac movements and breathing. It is easy to carry out 3D rebuilding of EUS images by a simple movement of shrinking the endoscope if radial echoendoscope EG 36 UR (Pentax Company, Hambourg, Germany) is used or by a rotational movement of 360° if the EG 38 UT (Pentax Company, Hambourg, Germany) is used.

Basic Principles of 3D US

There are 2 types of systems that have been developed, making use of either a series of 2D images produced by 1-dimensional (1D) or 2D arrays to produce 3D images directly. To avoid inaccuracies, 2 criteria must be met : the relative position and angulation of the acquired 2D images must be known accurately and the images must be

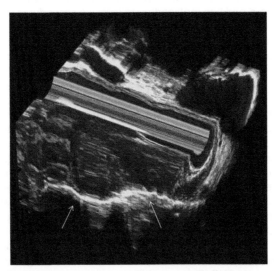

Fig. 4. A 3D reconstruction of an esophageal cancer UST4 (pleural involvement; *arrows*) using a radial electronic probe (PENTAX-EG 3670UR, Pentax Company, Hambourg Germany).

acquired rapidly and/or gated to avoid artifacts caused by respiratory, cardiac, and involuntary motion.

Tracked freehand systems

The operator holds an assembly composed of the transducer and an attachment and manipulates it over the anatomy. The 2D images are digitized as the transducer is moved while meeting 2 criteria: (1) the exact relative angulation and position of the ultrasound transducer must be known for each digitized image and (2) the operator must ensure that no significant gaps are left when scanning.

Three-dimensional reconstruction

The 3D reconstruction process refers to the generation of a 3D image from a digitized set of 2D images. The voxel-based volume approach was used. The 2D images are built into a 3D voxel-based volume (3D grid) by placing each digitized 2D image into its correct location in the volume. The main advantages were that no information was lost during the 3D reconstruction and a variety of rendering techniques were possible, but large data files are generated.

Visualization of 3D US images

The ability to visualize information in the 3D image depends critically on the rendering technique; 3 basic types are being used.

Surface-based viewing technique An operator or algorithm identifies the boundaries of structures to create a wireframe representation. These boundaries are shaded and illuminated so that surfaces, structures, or organs are visualized.

Multiplane viewing techniques
- Orthogonal views: 3 perpendicular planes are displayed simultaneously and can be moved or rotated.
- Polyhedron: the 3D images are presented as a multisided volume (polyhedron). The appropriate US image is painted on each face of the polyhedron, which can be manipulated.

Volume-based rendering techniques The 3D image is projected onto a 2D plane by casting rays through the 3D image. The voxel values intersected by each ray can be multiplied by factors and summed to produce different effects: multiplied by 1 and then added to form a radiograph-like image, multiplied by factors to produce translucency, or only the voxel is displayed with the maximum intensity along each ray.

Clinical Effect of 3D EUS

It is important to know the real effect of this new technique in studying human pathology. At present, the contribution of this new type of imagery is interesting only in tumoral pathology of the rectum. Indeed, the first studies on 3D EUS show that it is much easier to visualize the mesorectum and its limits in 3D echoendosopy than in 2D EUS (**Fig. 5**). This finding has an important effect on the therapeutic assumption of responsibility; it is known that the tumors of the rectum, which invade the quasi totality of the mesorectum (**Fig. 6**), have adverse outcomes resulting in metastatic rectal cancer. In addition, 3D echoendoscopy seems to have better reliability with endorectal EUS (ERUS) for the assessment of rectal cancer.[33] This finding was shown in several studies, particularly in the studies by Odegaard.[34] It would also seem that pancreatic 3D EUS makes it possible to better appreciate the tumoral infiltration on the level of the portosplenomesenteric confluence of pancreatic cancers (**Fig. 7**). There are still few data in the literature, but 2 series, that of Fritscher-Ravens[18]

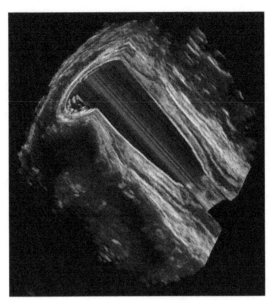

Fig. 5. A 3D reconstruction of normal rectum using a rigid radial probe (Hitachi RW 54, Hitachi Company, Tokyo, Japan).

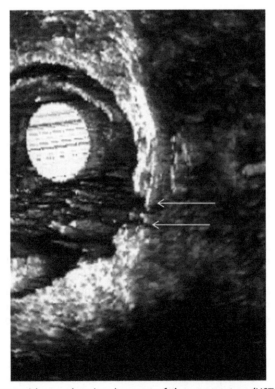

Fig. 6. Rectal cancer with complete involvement of the mesorectum (UST4) (*arrows*).

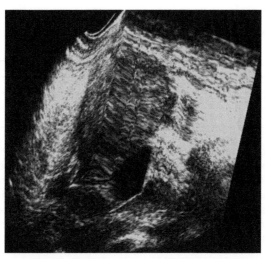

Fig. 7. Pancreatic cancer of the body of the pancreas with portal vein involvement. A 3D reconstruction using a linear probe (PENTAX-EG3870UTK, Pentax Company, Hambourg, Germany).

and Giovannini,[35] have the same conclusions that the assessment of venous extension would seem more precise in 3D pancreatic echoendoscopy. In conclusion, to date, it would seem that 3D EUS provides more information than conventional echoendoscopy about the level of cancers of the rectum. Other studies are necessary to specify the exact place of the 3D pancreatic echoendoscopy in the staging of pancreatic cancer.

THE AUTHOR'S EXPERIENCE IN 3D ERUS

Using this new software, thirty-five 3D ERUS examinations have been performed.[35] The indication of EUS was a local staging of rectal cancer in 35 cases. Before 3D ERUS scanning, a standard ERUS was performed. Then 3D rectal examination was performed using a radial electronic rigid probe. The 3D software was included in the new US scanning machine HITACHI 7500, 900, or Prerius and permits a reconstruction of the 2D EUS images in 6 different scans. Acquisition time is quick, around 10 to 25 seconds, and is a function of the number of images recorded.

Using 2D and 3D EUS, 35 rectal cancers were assessed. All tumors were located in the middle and lower part of the rectum, and stenotic tumors were excluded in this study. Performing a 3D EUS was possible in all cases. The 2D EUS data classified the tumors into T and N categories as follows: T1N0 (2 cases), T2N0 (3 cases), T3N0 (15 cases), T3N1 (12 cases), and T4N1 (3 cases). It was impossible using 2D images to precisely determine the degree of involvement of the mesorectum (more or less than 50%). No difference was showed using 3D ERUS for the superficial tumor (T1N0 and T2N0), but in 6 of 15 patients classified with T3N0 tumors, 3D ERUS showed malignant lymph nodes, which was confirmed surgically in 5 of 6 cases (**Table 1**).

On the other hand, 3D EUS allowed determination of the precise degree of infiltration of the mesorectum (see **Fig. 2**) in all cases and showed a quite complete invasion of it in 8 cases. These findings were confirmed in all cases by the surgical data. To summarize, 2D EUS assessed 25 of 35 (71.4%) rectal tumors correctly for T and N classification and 3D EUS improved this result to 31 of 35 (88.6%) correct evaluations.

Table 1 Correct findings using 3D ERUS	Rectal Cancer			
	T1N0/T2N0	T3N0	T3N1	T4N1
2D EUS	5	15	12	3
3D EUS	5	9	18	3
Surgical Findings	4	6	22	3

If the accuracy of 2D and 3D EUS in T staging is compared (T1–T2 vs T3–T4), there was no difference (34 of 35 accurate staging using the 2 techniques). But patients classified as 3D T3N0 (9 patients) developed less liver metastasis than those classified 2D T3N0 (15 patients) (1 of 9 vs 6 of 15, 11% vs 40%; $P = .002$). This difference was because 7 of 15 patients with 2D T3N0 rectal cancer had pT3N1 on the resected specimen. On the other hand, patients in whom 3D ERUS showed a large mesorectal infiltration 8 of 35 patients also developed more metastases (4 of 8 vs 7 of 27, 50% vs 26%; $P<.001$).

Santoro and colleagues[36] have evaluated the accuracy of high-resolution 3D EUS in distinguishing slight from massive submucosal invasion of early rectal tumors. A total of 142 consecutive patients with clinically possible pT1 rectal cancers underwent 3D EUS. Slight or massive irregularity of the hyperechoic submucosal layer was considered to characterize uT1-slight or uT1-massive tumors. Treatment was selected based on US findings; endoscopic resection or full-thickness transanal local excision was selected for uT1-slight lesions and radical resection was selected for uT1-massive tumors. US and histopathologic stagings were compared. In the final analyses, 126 patients were included. By 3D EUS 77 lesions were staged as uT0, 25 as uT1 slight, 20 as uT1 massive, and 4 as uT2. Histologically, adenomas were found in 75 patients, and tumor invasion was found in 44 lesions (24 pT1 slight, 16 pT1 massive, 4 pT2). The overall kappa score for the concordance between US and histopathologic stagings was 0.81 (95% confidence interval [CI], 0.72–0.89). No invasive carcinomas remained undetected. The depth of invasion was correctly determined in 87.2% of both pT1-slight and pT1-massive lesions. Considering the complete series of 126 patients, the accuracy of this modality in selecting appropriate management was 95.2% (kappa score 0.84; 95% CI, 0.71–0.96). Adequate surgery was performed in 87.5% cases of pT1 tumors. Imaging by 3D ERUS is useful for assessing the depth of submucosal invasion in early rectal cancer and selecting therapeutic options.

Summary

The 3D ERUS imaging with new software program, described in this article, is available at present and is easy to perform. Because there is no need for an external sensor mounted at the tip of the probe, manipulation of the rectal probe is facilitated. Imaging by 3D ERUS has a direct therapeutic effect on the pretherapeutic staging of rectal cancer and allows more precise definition of the mesorectal margins, with a direct effect on therapeutic decision making.

REFERENCES

1. Claudon M, Cosgrove D, Albrecht T, et al. Guidelines and good clinical practice recommendations for contrast enhanced ultrasound (CEUS)-update 2008. Ultraschall Med 2008;29:28–44.

2. Masaki T, Ohkawa S, Amano A, et al. Noninvasive assessment of tumor vascularity by contrast-enhanced ultrasonography and the prognosis of patients with nonresectable pancreatic carcinoma. Cancer 2005;103:1026–35.

3. Hocke M, Schulze E, Gottschalk P, et al. Contrast-enhanced endoscopic ultrasound in discrimination between focal pancreatitis and pancreatic cancer. World J Gastroenterol 2006;12:246–50.

4. Hintze RE, Adler A, Veltzke W, et al. Clinical significance of magnetic resonance cholangiopancreatography (MRCP) compared to endoscopic retrograde cholangiopancreatography (ERCP). Endoscopy 1997;29(3):182–7.

5. Domagk D, Wessling J, Reimer P, et al. Endoscopic retrograde cholangiopancreatography, intraductal ultrasonography, and magnetic resonance cholangiopancreatography in bile duct strictures: a prospective comparison of imaging diagnostics with histopathological correlation. Am J Gastroenterol 2004;99(9):1684–9.

6. Bhutani MS, Hoffman BJ, van Velse A, et al. Contrast-enhanced endoscopic ultrasonography with galactose microparticles:SHU508 A (Levovist). Endoscopy 1997;29(7):635–9.

7. Hirooka Y, Goto H, Ito A, et al. Contrast-enhanced endoscopic ultrasonography in pancreatic diseases: a preliminary study. Am J Gastroenterol 1998;93(4):632–5.

8. Becker D, Strobel D, Bernatik T, et al. Echo-enhanced color- and power-Doppler EUS for the discrimination between focal pancreatitis and pancreatic carcinoma. Gastrointest Endosc 2001;53(7):784–9.

9. Giovannini M. Endosonography: new developments in 2006. Scientific World Journal 2007;7:341–63 Gastroenterol; 89(11):2038–41.

10. Voss M, Hammel P, Molas G, et al. Value of endoscopic ultrasound guided fine needle aspiration biopsy in the diagnosis of solid pancreatic masses. Gut 2000;46(2):244–9.

11. Raut CP, Grau AM, Staerkel GA, et al. Diagnostic accuracy of endoscopic ultrasound-guided fine-needle aspiration in patients with presumed pancreatic cancer. J Gastrointest Surg 2003;7(1):118–26 [discussion: 127–8].

12. Giovannini M, Seitz JF, Monges G, et al. Fine-needle aspiration cytology guided by endoscopic ultrasonography: results in 141 patients. Endoscopy 1994;27(2):171–7.

13. Gress FG, Hawes RH, Savides TJ, et al. Endoscopic ultrasound-guided fine-needle aspiration biopsy using linear array and radial scanning endosonography. Gastrointest Endosc 1997;45(3):243–50.

14. Wiersema MJ, Vilmann P, Giovannini M, et al. Endosonography-guided fine-needle aspiration biopsy: diagnostic accuracy and complication assessment. Gastroenterology 1997;112(4):1087–95.

15. Chang KJ, Nguyen P, Erickson RA, et al. The clinical utility of endoscopic ultrasound-guided fine-needle aspiration in the diagnosis and staging of pancreatic carcinoma. Gastrointest Endosc 1997;45(5):387–93.

16. Williams DB, Sahai AV, Aabakken L, et al. Endoscopic ultrasound guided fine needle aspiration biopsy: a large single centre experience. Gut 1999;44(5):720–6.

17. Harewood GC, Wiersema MJ. Endosonography-guided fine needle aspiration biopsy in the evaluation of pancreatic masses. Am J Gastroenterol 2000;97(6):1386–91.

18. Fritscher-Ravens A, Brand L, Knofel WT, et al. Comparison of endoscopic ultrasound-guided fine needle aspiration for focal pancreatic lesions in patients with normal parenchyma and chronic pancreatitis. Am J Gastroenterol 2002;97(11):2768–75.

19. Kaufman AR, Sivak MV Jr. Endoscopic ultrasonography in the differential diagnosis of pancreatic disease. Gastrointest Endosc 1989;35(3):214–9.

20. Takeda K, Goto H, Hirooka Y, et al. Contrast-enhanced transabdominal ultrasonography in the diagnosis of pancreatic mass lesions. Acta Radiol 2003;44(1): 103–6.
21. Oshikawa O, Tanaka S, Ioka T, et al. Dynamic sonography of pancreatic tumors: comparison with dynamic CT. AJR Am J Roentgenol 2002;178(5): 1133–7.
22. Sofuni A, Iijima H, Moriyasu F, et al. Differential diagnosis of pancreatic tumors using ultrasound contrast imaging. J Gastroenterol 2005;40(5):518–25.
23. Nagase M, Furuse J, Ishii H, et al. Evaluation of contrast enhancement patterns in pancreatic tumors by coded harmonic sonographic imaging with a microbubble contrast agent. J Ultrasound Med 2003;22(8):789–95.
24. Kasono K, Hyodo T, Suminaga Y, et al. Contrast-enhanced endoscopic ultrasonography improves the preoperative localization of insulinomas. Endocr J 2002;49(4):517–22.
25. Rickes S, Unkrodt K, Ocran K, et al. Differentiation of neuroendocrine tumors from other pancreatic lesions by echo-enhanced power Doppler sonography and somatostatin receptor scintigraphy. Pancreas 2003;26(1):76–81.
26. Rosch T, Lightdale CJ, Botet JF, et al. Localization of pancreatic endocrine tumors by endoscopic ultrasonography. N Engl J Med 1992;326(26):1721–6.
27. Ueno N, Tomiyama T, Tano S, et al. Utility of endoscopic ultrasonography with color Doppler function for the diagnosis of islet cell tumor. Am J Gastroenterol 1996;91(4):772–6.
28. Itoh T, Hirooka Y, Itoh A, et al. Usefulness of contrast-enhanced transabdominal ultrasonography in the diagnosis of intraductal papillary mucinous tumors of the pancreas. Am J Gastroenterol 2005;100(1):144–52.
29. Fritscher-Ravens A, Sriram PV, Krause C, et al. Detection of pancreatic metastases by EUS-guided fine-needle aspiration. Gastrointest Endosc 2001;53(1): 65–70.
30. Flath B, Rickes S, Schweigert M, et al. Differentiation of a pancreatic metastasis of a renal cell carcinoma from a primary pancreatic carcinoma by echo-enhanced power Doppler sonography. Pancreatology 2003;3(4):349–51.
31. Hocke M, Menges M, Topalidis T, et al. Contrast-enhanced endoscopic ultrasound in discrimination between benign and malignant mediastinal and abdominal lymph nodes. J Cancer Res Clin Oncol 2008;134:473–80.
32. Kanamori A, Hirooka Y, Itoh A, et al. Usefulness of contrast-enhanced endoscopic ultrasonography in the differentiation between malignant and benign lymphadenopathy. Am J Gastroenterol 2006;101:45–51.
33. Kallimanis G, Garra BS, Tio TL. The feasibility of three-dimensional endoscopic ultrasonography: a preliminary report. Gastrointest Endosc 1995;41: 235–9.
34. Odegaard S, Nesje LB, Molin SO, et al. 3-D intraluminal sonography in the evaluation of gastrointestinal diseases. Abdom Imag 1999;24:449–51.
35. Giovannini M, Bories E, Pesenti C, et al. Three-dimensional endorectal ultrasound using a new freehand software program: results in 35 patients with rectal cancer. Endoscopy 2006;38(4):339–43.
36. Santoro GA, Gizzi G, Pellegrini L, et al. The value of high-resolution three-dimensional endorectal ultrasonography in the management of submucosal invasive rectal tumors. Dis Colon Rectum 2009;52(11):1837–43.

High-Definition and Filter-Aided Colonoscopy

Jenny Sauk, MD[a], Arthur Hoffman, MD[b],
Sharmila Anandasabapathy, MD[a], Ralf Kiesslich, MD, PhD[b],*

KEYWORDS

• Colonoscopy • High definition • Filter technologies • Adenoma

Recent concerns that the protective effect of colonoscopy is lower than previously thought have shifted attention to improving the precision of colonoscopy.[1–6] Although efforts at optimizing the quality of colonoscopies are ongoing, a pooled adenoma detection miss rate of 22% (15%–32%) in tandem colonoscopy studies by experienced endoscopists and increasing recognition of nonpolypoid flat premalignant lesions, have lead to accelerated interest in technological developments to improve adenoma detection and assist in the characterization of premalignant lesions.[7,8]

The prognosis for patients with malignancies of the lower gastrointestinal (GI) tract is strictly dependent on early detection of premalignant and malignant lesions. Three steps are important for a proper endoscopic diagnosis: recognition, characterization, and confirmation. Computer and chip technologies have faced major technological advances that can improve endoscopic diagnostics. High-resolution or high-definition (HD) endoscopes can improve *recognition* or detection of lesions of the colon. Chromoendoscopy or filter-aided colonoscopy (virtual chromoendoscopy) can enhance *characterization* of lesion morphology and surface architecture to better predict histology. Finally, conventional or in vivo histology (confocal laser endomicroscopy) can provide histologic *confirmation* to define whether neoplastic changes are present or not.

HIGH-DEFINITION COLONOSCOPY

The resolution of an endoscopic image is different from magnification, and is defined as the ability to distinguish between 2 points that are close together. High-resolution imaging improves the ability to discriminate details while magnification enlarges the image. In digital video imaging, resolution is a function of pixel density. Through

[a] The Henry D. Janowitz Division of Gastroenterology, Mount Sinai School of Medicine, 1 Gustave Levy Place, Box 1069, New York, NY 10029, USA
[b] I Med Klinik, Universitätsmedizin Mainz Langenbeckstr 1, 55131 Mainz, Germany
* Corresponding author.
E-mail address: Kiesslich@uni-mainz.de

Gastroenterol Clin N Am 39 (2010) 859–881
doi:10.1016/j.gtc.2010.08.022
0889-8553/10/$ – see front matter © 2010 Published by Elsevier Inc.

gastro.theclinics.com

high-pixel density charged-coupled devices (CCD), high-resolution endoscopes provide slightly magnified views of the GI tract but with greater mucosal detail. Magnification endoscopy uses a movable lens controlled by the endoscopist to vary the degree of magnification, which ranges from 1.5× to 150×. Newly designed magnification endoscopes provide both high-resolution and magnification features.

More recently, HD endoscopes are available. CCDs convert light information into an electronic signal. This signal is processed into an image via the video processor. The standard analog broadcasting systems (Phase Alternate Line [PAL] and National Television System Committee [NTSC]) generate approximately 480 to 576 scanning lines on a screen. Now, the new HD endoscopes can generate up to 1080 scanning lines on a screen, which further increases the resolution. Surface analysis on distinct lesions can be performed even before magnification.

High-Definition Colonoscopy for the Detection of Colorectal Neoplasia

Theoretically, the effectiveness of endoscopy should depend on the resolution. The better the image quality, the more likely it should be to obtain the right diagnosis. Rex and colleagues[9] called for further evaluation of high-definition endoscopy for adenoma detection when they noted a high number of subjects with greater than or equal to 1 adenoma regardless of whether they were randomized to withdrawal with white light using HD endoscopes or narrow band imaging (67% vs 65%; p = ns). It was unclear whether high adenoma detection rates in this study were caused by improved visualization from HD endoscopes or simply precise withdrawal technique from an experienced operator. However, the few dedicated studies subsequently evaluating the effectiveness of HD endoscopy over standard resolution (SR) endoscopy in adenoma detection have been conflicting. **Table 1** summarizes the recent published data.

Table 1
High-definition versus standard colonoscopy for the detection of colorectal adenomas

Author	Year	Design	N	Primary Outcome	HD	SR	Outcome
East et al[10]	2008	Prospective, cohort study	130	Subjects with at least 1 adenoma	71%	60%	Not significant
Pellisé et al[11]	2008	Prospective, randomized controlled	620	Mean number of adenomas per subject	0.43	0.45	Not significant
Tribonias et al[12]	2010	Prospective randomized	390	Polyp detection rate per subject	1.76	1.31	P = .03 (no difference for adenoma detection)
Burke et al[13]	2010	Retrospective, comparative cohort study	852	Polyp detection rate	39.9%	36.9%	Not significant
Buchner et al[14]	2010	Retrospective study	2430	Adenoma detection rate	28.8%	24.3%	P = .012
Hoffman et al[15]	2010	Prospective, randomized controlled	200	Subjects with at least 1 adenoma	38%	13%	P<.0001

Several studies suggest that high-definition colonoscopy is *not* significantly better than SR colonoscopy at improving adenoma detection. East and colleagues[10] compared adenoma detection rates using HD colonoscopy versus SR colonoscopy in a prospective cohort study of 130 subjects where colonoscopy was performed by 1 experienced endoscopist using optimal withdrawal techniques. This study revealed no significant difference in adenoma detection rates (71% vs 60%; P = .20), number of proximal hyperplastic polyps (31 vs 23; P = .35), and number of overall adenomas detected (93 vs 88; P = .12) between the two technologies, respectively. However, for small (<6 mm), nonflat adenomas, a significantly higher number of lesions were detected with HD (P = .03). They concluded that high-quality withdrawal techniques in both groups may have been the most important factor contributing to high adenoma detection rates in both SR and HD colonoscopy.

In a randomized, controlled trial including 620 subjects, Pellisé and colleagues[11] also investigated whether HD colonoscopy was more effective in adenoma detection than SR colonoscopy by a group of 7 full-time gastroenterologists who spent more than 50% of their time performing procedures. Both techniques detected a similar number of adenomas on a per-subject analysis (HD 0.43 vs SR 0.45; p = ns), with no differences in the type of lesions detected, distribution of lesions along the colon, the degree of dysplasia, or morphology of the adenomas. Even in standard practice conditions, HD colonoscopy did not detect significantly more colorectal neoplasia than SR colonoscopy.

In a smaller prospective study, Tribonias and colleagues[12] did note a significantly increased polyp detection rate per subject in the HD versus SR colonoscopy group (1.76 vs 1.31; P = .03). However, the adenoma detection rate did not differ significantly in the two groups.[12] Similarly, Burke and colleagues[13] powered their comparative retrospective cohort study of 852 subjects to detect a 10% difference in polyp detection between HD and SR colonoscopy and yielded negative results. However, they showed that HD improved the detection of subjects with greater than or equal to 3–6-mm or smaller adenomas (P = .050).

Two more recent studies have shown that HD colonoscopy *can* improve overall adenoma detection. Although retrospective, the study by Buchner and colleagues[14] is the largest to date with 2430 nonselected subjects in a general practice setting by various endoscopists. Not only was there a statistically significant increase in polyp detection (HD 42.2% vs SD 37.8%; P = .026) but also adenoma detection, (HD 28.8% vs SR 24.3%; P = .012) even after adjusting for potential confounding factors. Once again, the highest polyp detection with HD occurred in polyps 0 to 5 mm in size, (HD 32.3% vs SR 27.2%; P = .009). In a smaller prospective study, Hoffman and colleagues[15] also showed that HD colonoscopy is superior in adenoma detection and in identifying significantly more patients with at least 1 adenoma.

HD deserves further study to clarify its clinical value. Many of the studies have suggested that there is increased detection of diminutive adenomas (1–5 mm) with this technology. Because diminutive lesions can harbor unfavorable histology, the detection and removal of these lesions may be clinically important.[16–18] However, the value of detecting and removing diminutive adenomas (1–5 mm) still remains unclear. Regardless of conflicting data, the transition from standard resolution to high-definition endoscopy is likely inevitable; endoscopists prefer high definition because they simply see better and there is no learning curve for its use.

Chromoendoscopy Technique

Chromoendoscopy or tissue staining is an old endoscopic technique that has been used for decades. It involves the topical application of stains or pigments to improve localization, characterization, or diagnosis of a lesion. It is a useful adjunct to endoscopy; the contrast between normally stained and abnormally stained epithelium enables the endoscopist to make a diagnosis or to direct biopsies based on a specific reaction or enhancement of surface morphology.

The technique for staining is simple and easy to learn. Chromoendoscopy can be done in an untargeted fashion of the whole colon (panchromoendoscopy) or directed toward a specific lesion (targeted staining). While spraying dyes in the colon in an untargeted fashion, the endoscopist needs to direct the endoscope and catheter tip toward the colorectal mucosa and use a combination of rotational clockwise-counter clockwise movements with simultaneous withdrawal of the endoscope tip. The movements are necessary to achieve an even spread of the dye on the mucosa.

Contrast dyes, which coat the colonic mucosa, include 0.1% to 0.4% indigo carmine. This dye has been used for most studies of chromoendoscopy in the colon. The dye is not absorbed but simply highlights surface topography by pooling in grooves caused by mucosal lesions. In addition, 0.1% methylene blue has been used in colonoscopy and is an absorptive dye actively taken up by normal epithelial cells in the colon and small intestine. There has been some suggestion that methylene blue can cause oxidative DNA damage in cells exposed to white light (WL) during chromoendoscopy.[19,20] However, a recent study did not show an increase in cancers in subjects who underwent chromoendoscopy with methylene blue.[21]

Chromoendoscopy for improved adenoma detection

Although individual authors drew different conclusions regarding the effectiveness of chromoendoscopy over conventional colonoscopic examinations for adenoma detection, a recent Cochrane review pooled the overall experience with chromoendoscopy for adenoma detection from 4 prospective, randomized trials in subjects without inflammatory bowel disease or polyposis syndromes (**Table 2**).[22–28] Despite nonsignificant adenoma detection rates in 3 of the 4 studies, when pooled together, the studies revealed that chromoendoscopy yields more subjects with at least 1 neoplastic lesion (odds ratio [OR]: 1.61 [95% confidence interval (CI) 1.24–2.09]) and more subjects with 3 or more neoplastic lesions (OR 2.55 [95% CI 1.49–4.36]) than standard colonoscopy.[23–26] The review authors concluded that there is

> strong evidence that chromoendoscopy enhances the detection of neoplasia in the colon and rectum. Patients with neoplastic polyps, particularly those with multiple polyps, are at increased risk of developing colorectal cancer. Such lesions, which presumably would be missed with conventional colonoscopy, could contribute to the interval cancer numbers on any surveillance program.[22]

A more recent multicenter study conducted in the United States randomized 50 subjects with a history of colorectal cancer or adenomas to tandem colonoscopy with the second examination as standard colonoscopy or chromoendoscopy.[29] This study found that the second chromoendoscopy detected adenomas in more subjects than did intensive 20-minute inspection with a second standard colonoscopy (44% vs 17%), changing management in 27% of subjects who would have been classified as free of adenomas. Similar to the Lapalus study, the majority of adenomas detected were significantly smaller (2.66 mm ± 0.97 mm) and right sided.

Despite increasing polyp and adenoma detection with chromoendoscopy, studies have repeatedly demonstrated a longer withdrawal time.[22,23,26,27] Although withdrawal techniques differed in the 4 studies included in the Cochrane review, withdrawal time was longer in the chromoendoscopy group (3–75 minutes) than with the control group (2–60 minutes).[22] In the Stoffel study, despite the 20-minute intensive inspection in the

Table 2
Chromoendoscopy versus standard colonoscopy for adenoma detection

Author	Year	N	Primary Outcome	Chromo	Standard	Outcome
Brooker et al[23]	2002	259	Total number of adenomas	125	49	Not significant
Hurlstone et al[25]	2004	260	Subjects with ≥3 adenomas	13	4	P<.01
Le Rhun et al[24]	2006	198	Total number of adenomas per subject	0.6	0.5 (HRC)	Not significant
Lapalus et al[26]	2006	292	Subjects with ≥1 adenoma	40%	36% (HRC)	Not significant
Brown et al[22] (Cochrane Review)	2007	1009	a) Subjects with ≥1 adenoma b) Subjects with ≥3 adenoma	a) OR in favor of chromo: 1.6 b) OR in favor of chromo: 2.55		95% CI: 1.24– 2.09 95% CI: 1.49–4.36
Stoffel et al[29]	2008	50	Adenomas per subject on second examination	0.7	0.2	P<.01

Abbreviations: CI, confidence interval; HRC, high-resolution colonoscopy; OR, odds ratio.

standard colonoscopy arm, chromoendoscopy still required more time than intensive inspection, (36.9 vs 27.3 minutes; $P<.01$).[29]

Several studies have attempted different methods of staining to improve procedure time and to maintain high adenoma detection rates with chromoendoscopy. As attention has focused on flat or diminutive, right-sided lesions, Park and colleagues[30] randomized 316 consecutive subjects to a repeat examination of the ascending colon and cecum only with a second colonoscopy or chromoendoscopy with indigo carmine. During the second diagnostic intubation, 17.4% of subjects in the chromoendoscopy group and 5.3% in the standard colonoscopy group had at least 1 adenoma ($P<.001$). There was no statistically significant difference in procedural time between the two groups as chromoendoscopy only occurred in the ascending colon and cecum and standard colonoscopy was fixed to at least 120 seconds of inspection time. If the clinically significant flat adenomas are mainly right sided, this method of focusing examination to the ascending colon and cecum could increase diagnostic yield of adenomas without adding the procedural burden of staining the entire colon.

However, Hurlstone and colleagues[25] randomized 260 subjects to panchromoendoscopy or targeted chromoendoscopy and discovered that although extubation times did not significantly differ between the groups (Chromo [median 17 minutes] vs targeted [median 15 minutes]), in the panchromoendoscopy group, more adenomas were detected ($P<.05$), more diminutive (<4mm) adenomas were detected overall ($P = .03$), and most importantly, more flat and diminutive adenomas were detected in the right colon ($P<.05$). This study suggests that panchromoendoscopy is better for improved adenoma detection than targeted chromoendoscopy. Nevertheless, chromoendoscopy is still regarded as cumbersome and time intensive and has not been widely incorporated into everyday practice.

Diminutive adenomas contributed most to the higher adenoma detection with chromoendoscopy in the majority of the studies.[23–30] As previously mentioned, the significance of these diminutive adenomas require further investigation, but if recent data suggesting that 7% to 15% of small adenomas (5–10mm) show advanced histology, further optical enhancements, such as chromoendoscopy, should be routinely adopted in clinical practice.[16–18]

Chromoendoscopy for improved characterization

In addition to increased detection, chromoendoscopy has been evaluated for its characterization abilities. Surface analysis of stained colorectal lesions was a new optical impression for the endoscopists in the 1990s. First, Kudo and colleagues[31] described that some of the regular staining patterns are often seen in hyperplastic polyps or normal mucosa; whereas, unstructured surface architecture was associated with malignancy. Also, adenomas can be classified better (tubular vs villous) upon detailed inspection. This experience has lead to a categorization of the different staining patterns in the colon: The so-called pit-pattern classification differentiated 5 types and several subtypes. Types 1 and 2 are staining patterns predicting non-neoplastic lesions; whereas, types 3 to 5 are predicting neoplastic lesions. With the help of this classification, the endoscopist may predict histology with good accuracy.

Axelrad and colleagues first reported a sensitivity and specificity of chromoendoscopy of 95% and 93%, respectively, with a diagnostic accuracy of 81%, but the ability of chromoendoscopy to differentiate between adenomatous polyps from non-adenomatous polyps have varied considerably in several large studies using indigo carmine with sensitivity and specificity between 82% to 98% and 52% to 95%, respectively (**Table 3**).[32–41]

Table 3
Chromoendoscopy for polyp characterization

Author	Year	Design	N	Outcome	Sensitivity (%)	Specificity (%)	Overall Accuracy (%)
Axelrad et al[36]	1996	Prospective study; lesion analysis	36	High-resolution, magnifying Chromo polyp analysis	95	93	81
Togashi et al[37]	1999	Prospective study; lesion analysis	1280	Magnifying chromo polyp analysis	92.0	73.3	88.4
Tung et al[38]	2001	Prospective study; lesion analysis	141	Magnifying chromo polyp analysis	93.8	64.6	80.1
Eisen et al[39]	2002	Prospective, multicenter trial; lesion analysis	299	High-resolution, Chromo polyp analysis	82	82	88
Konishi et al[40]	2003	Prospective, randomized study	660	Standard chromo vs Magnifying chromo	SC: 90 MC: 97	SC: 61 MC: 100	SC: 68 MC:92
Fu et al[33]	2004	Prospective study; lesion analysis	122	Conventional colonoscopy vs Chromo vs Magnifying chromo	CC: 88.8 C: 93.1 MC:96.3	CC: 93.1 C: 76.1 MC:93.5	CC: 84.0 C: 89.3 MC: 95.6
Su et al[35]	2004	Prospective study; lesion analysis	230	Magnifying chromo polyp analysis	95.1	86.8	91.9

Abbreviations: C, chromo colonoscopy; CC, conventional colonoscopy; MC, magnifying chromo; N, NBI.

Magnifying chromoendoscopy can increase the diagnostic accuracy even further. Konishi and colleagues[40] randomized 660 subjects to standard chromoendoscopy with 0.2% indigo carmine and magnifying chromoendoscopy in a prospective fashion to determine the surface staining pattern (pit-pattern classification) and predict the malignant potential of lesions. Magnifying endoscopes significantly improved diagnostic accuracy (92%) as compared with chromoendoscopy with standard video endoscopes (68%).

Although interobserver and intraobserver variability among experienced endoscopists for determining pit pattern is good ($\kappa = 0.72$; $\kappa = 0.81$, respectively), chromoendoscopy is still not widely used in clinical practice for the characterization of lesions.[42] Once again, the time-intensive nature of chromoendoscopy may limit its use, but the question remains whether more readily available high-definition or high-resolution endoscopes may help with determining pit patterns without the use of magnifying endoscopes. In one study, 150 subjects undergoing high-resolution screening colonoscopy were evaluated for polyps less than 5mm in the rectum and sigmoid colon.[43] The sensitivity and specificity for predicting non-neoplastic polyps only minimally improved from 93% to 94% and 60% to 64%, respectively, with the addition of indigo carmine. As high-definition and high-resolution colonoscopes are more convenient to use and more readily available, studies should evaluate whether this technology can help characterize lesions as well as magnifying chromoendoscopy.

Chromoendoscopy in high-risk populations

Hereditary nonpolyposis colorectal cancer Given the fast progression of hereditary nonpolyposis colorectal cancer (HNPCC) syndrome lesions to cancer, with data showing 4 out of 11 interval cancers within 3.5 years of normal colonoscopic assessment, patients with HNPCC syndrome might benefit from enhanced endoscopic imaging to help detect flat and depressed lesions.[44,45] Three tandem colonoscopy studies sought to discover the potentially added benefit of chromoendoscopy in this high-risk patient population. Among 25 asymptomatic subjects with HNPCC in Hurlstone's study, targeted chromoendoscopy identified 24 lesions in 13 subjects, but panchromoendoscopy helped detect 52 more lesions in 16 subjects, with more adenomas detected in the panchromoendoscopy group ($P = .001$).[46] Lecomte and colleagues[47] also found significantly more adenomas on the second chromoendoscopy examination of the proximal colon than on the first examination. Stoffel and colleagues[48] went on further to say that the second examination itself with white light lead to higher adenoma detection with minimal contribution from chromoendoscopy. Because the study was small and not powered to detect a difference in adenoma detection between intensive inspection on second examination and chromoendoscopy, future multicenter trials may need to look into adenoma detection rates with not only chromoendoscopy but other enhancing imaging modalities.

Ulcerative colitis Patients with ulcerative colitis (UC) have a significantly higher risk for the development of colitis-associated colorectal cancer, with a reported cumulative incidence rate of colorectal cancer that is 2.5% at 20 years, 7.6% at 30 years, and 10.8% at 40 years, with higher rates if patients have primary sclerosing cholangitis.[49,50] Accepted guidelines call for 2 to 4 random biopsies every 10 cm of the colon to look for dysplastic changes. Despite this, 16 of 30 cancers are interval cancers for patients already in surveillance programs.[51] With growing knowledge that dysplastic changes are subtle yet visible, we need new methods to improve our targeted biopsies.[52]

A large study using magnifying chromoendoscopy in 886 subjects with UC found that dysplasia and early cancer were characterized by granular or nodular protruding mucosa or by lowly protruding or flat mucosa, often associated with redness.[53] Dye-spraying endoscopy was useful for detection of all lesions with intraepithelial neoplasias characterized by a staining pattern III-V (**Fig. 1**). Dysplasia was never found in normal-looking mucosa after staining. Thus, enhanced imaging could potentially improve the detection of these visible lesions. Random biopsies are still widely performed but cannot eradicate the fear of overlooked cancers.

In 2003, the first randomized, controlled trial was published to test whether chromo and magnifying endoscopy might facilitate early detection of intraepithelial neoplasia in patients with ulcerative colitis.[54] A total of 165 subjects with long-standing ulcerative colitis were randomized at a 1:1 ratio to undergo conventional colonoscopy or colonoscopy with chromoendoscopy using 0.1% methylene blue. Lesions in the colon were evaluated according to a modified pit-pattern classification, (pit-pattern I-II: endoscopic prediction non-neoplastic; pit-pattern III-V: endoscopic prediction neoplastic). In the chromoendoscopy group, there was a significantly better correlation between endoscopic assessment of degree and extent of colonic inflammation and histopathologic findings compared with the conventional colonoscopy group. More targeted biopsies were possible, and significantly more intraepithelial neoplasias were detected in the chromoendoscopy group (32 vs 10). Furthermore, using the modified pit-pattern classification and chromoendoscopy, both the sensitivity and specificity for differentiation between non-neoplastic and neoplastic lesions were 93%. In a subsequent study, chromoendoscopy with confocal endomicroscopy increased

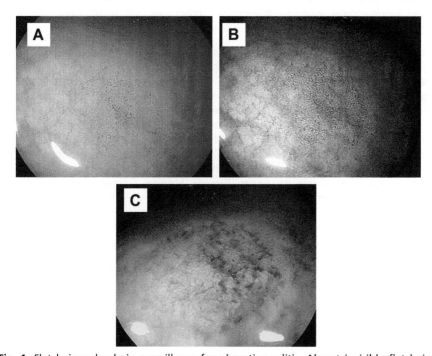

Fig. 1. Flat lesion: dysplasia surveillance for ulcerative colitis. Almost invisible flat lesion during ulcerative colitis surveillance. (*A*) Examination under high-definition white light. (*B*) I-scan with surface enhancement and vessel enhancement facilitates the recognition of subtle changes. (*C*) Chromoendoscopy with methylene blue unmasks a well-defined circumscribed lesion with tubular IIIL pit pattern suggestive of colitis-associated dysplasia. Target biopsy or endoscopic removal is recommended.

the diagnostic yield of intraepithelial neoplasia 4.75 fold as compared with conventional colonoscopy and biopsy techniques.[55]

Hurlstone detected the intraepithelial neoplasia detection rate from targeted biopsies to be 8% (49 of 644) versus 0.16% (20 of 12,850) from nontargeted biopsies, suggesting that the random biopsies are low yield. Among 350 subjects with UC, magnifying chromoendoscopy yielded 69 lesions compared with only 24 with standard colonoscopy.[56] Rutter and colleagues[57] similarly found no dysplastic tissue in 2904 nontargeted biopsies, and detected 9 dysplastic lesions in 157 targeted biopsies using chromoendoscopy. More recently, Marion and colleagues found that with targeted chromoendoscopy, increased number of biopsies confirmed low- and high-grade dysplastic tissue [16 and 1], respectively, than random biopsies [3 and 0]; (p = 0.001) and targeted non-dye spray colonoscopy [8 and 1]; (p = 0.057).[58]

Taken together, these data suggest that targeted biopsies after dye staining will replace random biopsies in the future.[53–59] Magnifying chromoendoscopy is a valid tool for better endoscopic detection of intraepithelial neoplasia in patients with long-standing ulcerative colitis and an increased ability to differentiate non-neoplastic from neoplastic lesions. A recent Medical Position Statement of the American Gastro-enterological Association endorsed the use of chromoendoscopy in the surveillance of patients with UC for physicians who have expertise with this technique.[60] The European consensus guidelines even adopted the concept of smart biopsies of lesions detected and analyzed by chromoendoscopy as an alternative to untargeted quadrant biopsies of apparently normal mucosa after chromoendoscopy.[61] Future studies should longitudinally evaluate if improved outcomes will result from improved dysplasia detection in patients with ulcerative colitis.

Digital chromoendoscopy Despite increased dysplasia detection in higher-risk patient populations with chromoendoscopy and increased adenoma and polyp detection rates for the general population, it is not widely used in clinical practice because of the cumbersome nature of the dye spray. As a result, digital modalities have developed to provide enhanced chromoendoscopy images without the use of dye. Conventional white-light endoscopy uses the full, visible wave-length range to produce a red-green-blue image. New filter technologies can narrow red-green-blue bands (ie, narrow band imaging [NBI]) to enhance microvessel architecture or use adaptive image postprocessing algorithms (filtering and logic) to segment and extract image irregularities (ie, i-scan [Pentax Medical Company, Montvale, NJ, USA]; Fujinon Intelligent Color Enhancement system [FICE], [Fujinon, Inc, Wayne, NJ, USA]) (**Fig. 2**). This technology can modulate different forms of enhancement, which leads to an accentuation of the vasculature, the surface architecture, or the pattern visualization.

NBI
NBI uses endoscopic light with a shorter wavelength to enhance superficial mucosal capillaries and mucosal surface patterns. Greater absorption of illuminating bands by hemoglobin will cause the blood vessels to look darker. The resulting images look like chromoendoscopy without dyes. By highlighting the aberrant microvessel architecture and mucosal surface patterns in adenomas, NBI *should* improve adenoma detection further.

NBI for adenoma detection However, 5 randomized trials with mixed subject populations (screening and diagnostic colonoscopy) suggest that for the average-risk population, NBI does not improve adenoma detection (**Table 4**).[9,62,63] In one study, adenoma detection rates were high in the control groups with minimal added benefit

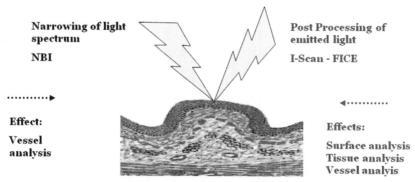

Fig. 2. Digital chromoendoscopy. Digital chromoendoscopy can be achieved by simply pressing a button on the endoscope. NBI focuses on vessel architecture by narrowing the light spectrum, which is emitted to the mucosa. FICE and i-scan are technologies that use the reflected light for postprocessing light filtering, which is used to obtain different effects (eg, surface, tissue, and vessel enhancement).

upon addition of NBI.[9] Kaltenbach and colleagues also did not find a significant difference in adenoma detection rates between WL and NBI use (44% vs 50%; p = ns) and state the same reasoning of high detection rates in the WL arm for not showing a diagnostic benefit with NBI use.[62]

Adler and colleagues[63] in a large multicenter prospective, randomized trial of 1256 subjects and 6 endoscopists, did not find a difference in adenoma detection between the two groups (0.32 vs 0.34) and the total number of adenomas (200 vs 216), even with a small but significantly prolonged withdrawal time (8.5 vs 7.9 minutes; $P<.05$). Hyperplastic polyps were more frequently detected in the NBI group ($P = .03$), but similar to the study by East and colleagues,[10,63] flat adenomas were detected more frequently in the control group, with the investigators speculating that the image environment with NBI may have been too dark to image the subtle lesions. In a preliminary study by this same group, the adenoma detection rate in the WL arm increased over time from 8.0% to 26.5%, with the rate of the NBI arm being unchanged. The investigators questioned whether a learning effect from the NBI imaging improved recognition for lesions in white light.[64]

A more recent prospective, randomized trial including subjects with positive immunologic fecal occult blood tests were randomly assigned to NBI versus WL during the withdrawal phase. A total of 201 and 198 ($P = .69$) adenomas were noted in the NBI and WL group, respectively. High rates of adenomas were detected in both groups (WL 58.3% and NBI 57.3%). HD imaging in the WL group may have contributed to the high adenoma detection rates reported here.[65] Contrary to the findings in Adler's study, flat adenomas were detected more frequently in NBI than in WL (21.4% vs 9.3%; $P = .019$), with flat adenomas representing 11% of total adenomas diagnosed. The investigators argued for a potential role of NBI in the detection of flat lesions, but more studies are necessary to understand the role of NBI in this subgroup.

Only Inoue and colleagues[66] reported more adenomas, especially diminutive adenomas ($P<.05$), in the pan-colonic NBI group. However, of 243 subjects, the percentage of subjects with at least 1 adenoma or multiple adenomas did not differ significantly between the standard colonoscopy and pan-colonic NBI group. Furthermore, most of the NBI was being performed by 1 endoscopist, possibly biasing the results toward a higher adenoma detection rate in the NBI group in this study. Future

Table 4
NBI for adenoma detection

Author	Year	Design	N	Primary Outcome	NBI	Standard	Outcome
Rex et al[9]	2007	Prospective, randomized study	434	% subjects with ≥1 adenoma	65%	67% (HD)	Not significant
Kaltenbach et al[62]	2008	Prospective, randomized study: randomized first scope; tandem colonoscopy	276	Neoplasm miss rate (neoplasms missed/ all subjects per group)	12.6%	12.1% (HD)	Not significant
Inoue et al[66]	2008	Prospective, randomized study	243	a) % subjects with ≥1 adenoma b) Total number adenomas	a) 42% b) 102	a) 34% b) 65	a) Not significant b) $P = .046$
Adler et al[63]	2009	Prospective, multicenter, randomized study	1256	Adenoma detection rate (all adenomas/all participants)	0.32	0.34 (HD)	Not significant
Paggi et al[65]	2009	Prospective, randomized study	211	% subjects with ≥1 adenoma	57.3%	58.3% (HD)	Not significant

Abbreviation: HD, high definition.

studies should focus on high-risk groups, the role of NBI in detecting flat/depressed, diminutive and hyperplastic lesions, and the significance of these lesions.

High-risk populations

HNPCC One of the high-risk states that have been studied using NBI is Lynch syndrome (HNPCC). In a tandem colonoscopy study, East and colleagues detected more lesions on NBI after first pass WLE, with an increased number of adenomas detected from 25 before NBI to 46 after NBI (p<0.001).[67] The authors concluded that for high-risk groups, patients may benefit from NBI colonoscopy.

On the other hand, Huneburg and colleagues[68] reported detecting more adenomas through chromoendoscopy than NBI or standard white light in subjects with HNPCC, with at least 1 adenoma found in 15% of subjects by both standard and NBI compared with 28% of subjects with chromoendoscopy.

Ulcerative colitis In ulcerative colitis, the role of NBI is not as promising. Dekker and colleagues[69] used a prototype NBI system to compare NBI versus standard resolution white light colonoscopy to detect neoplasia in subjects with longstanding ulcerative colitis. All subjects underwent 2 colonoscopies within 3 weeks between the two examinations: one with NBI with targeted biopsies and one with standard colonoscopy with random biopsy specimens with a randomized order in which they would receive the procedures. Although twice as many lesions were detected with NBI than WL, the increase in targeted biopsies did not translate to a higher dysplasia detection rate in the NBI group. WL detected more neoplastic lesions than NBI (12 vs 9) and both WL and NBI only identified 8 out of the 12 subjects with neoplasia, corresponding to a sensitivity of 67%. Because both strategies failed to detect neoplasia in 4 subjects, with a miss rate of 33% for each strategy, the investigators argued that a random biopsy protocol cannot be abandoned in favor of NBI. The investigators called for future studies using brighter, newer NBI technology because the dark images on the prototype may have contributed to the low sensitivity in the NBI group.

Two other studies have looked at NBI use in ulcerative colitis to detect neoplastic lesions. Matsumoto and colleagues[70] classified visible protruding lesions by NBI and flat areas of the colon. A total of 296 areas were considered suspicious by NBI (20 protruded lesions, 276 flat mucosa). The sensitivity, specificity, and overall accuracy of NBI to detect a neoplastic region was 80.0%, 84.2%, and 84.1%.

Van den Broek and colleagues[71] also tested the ability of NBI to detect neoplastic lesions and had equally disappointing results. Subjects were randomized to white light endoscopy, NBI, and autofluorescence. Sixteen neoplastic lesions and 82 non-neoplastic lesions were included for an overall sensitivity, specificity, and accuracy of NBI of 75%, 81%, and 80%, respectively. East and colleagues[72] believe that because of background inflammation in colitis, NBI may not be able to improve visualization of hyper vascular dysplastic lesions.

NBI for characterization of lesions Although data in favor of NBI for adenoma detection is poor, data for characterization of lesions with NBI show more promise. Several studies have used analysis of mucosal pit pattern and vascular pattern (ie, brown hue, dense vessels, vascular pattern intensity) to assess risk of neoplasia risk of a lesion (**Fig. 3**).[73–80]

In the first pilot study with NBI for colorectal lesions, Machida and colleagues[81] point out that the narrow band imaging system provides imaging features additional to

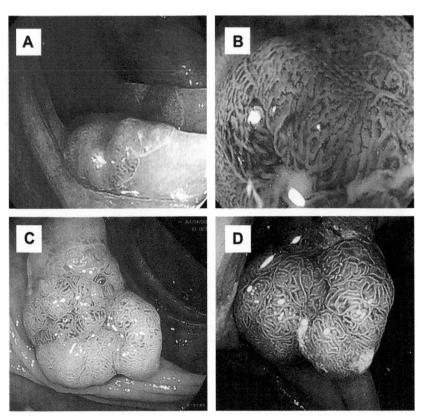

Fig. 3. Flat lesion with high-definition white light, NBI, and i-scan. Flat lesion via (*A*) high-definition white light. (*B*) NBI: brown vascular pattern; Kudo pit pattern IIIL: tubularlike pit pattern suggestive of adenomatous lesion. (*C*) I-scan with surface enhancement, villous surface pattern (pit pattern IV). (*D*) I-scan with surface enhancement and vessel characterization.

those of both conventional endoscopy and chromoendoscopy with a sensitivity and specificity for detecting neoplastic lesions comparable to chromoendoscopy of 100% and 75%, respectively.

One systematic review pooled the results from 6 studies, including the Machida study, to determine the sensitivity, specificity, and overall accuracy with NBI in determining neoplastic lesions.[73–76,81–83] NBI distinguished a total of 358 neoplastic lesions from 158 nonneoplastic lesions in these 6 studies with a pooled sensitivity of 92% (89%–94%), specificity of 86% (80%–91%), and an overall accuracy (95% CI) of 89% (87%–91%).[82] Five of the 6 studies provided information on chromoendoscopy as well with comparable sensitivity (91% [83%–96%]), specificity, (89% [83%–93%]) and overall accuracy (91% [85%–94%]) to NBI (**Table 5**).[73,74,76,81,83] For distinguishing neoplasms from non-neoplastic lesions, NBI appears equivalent to chromoendoscopy.

More recently, with the high accuracy of NBI in determining neoplastic lesions, studies are looking at the ability to make an NBI-based optical diagnosis of small colorectal polyps without formal histopathology. In one study, 4 colonoscopists with different levels of experience predicted polyp histology using optical diagnosis with

Table 5
NBI for adenoma characterization

Author	Year	Design	N	NBI Classification	Sensitivity	Specificity	Overall Accuracy
Machida et al[81]	2004	Prospective comparative study; polyp analysis	34	Kudo classification	CC: 85.3% Chromo: 100% NBI: 100%	CC: 44.4% Chromo: 75% NBI: 75%	CC: 79.1% Chromo: 93.4% NBI: 93.4%
Su et al[74]	2006	Prospective comparative study; polyp analysis	78	Brownish vascular pattern	CC: 82.9% Chromo: 95.7% NBI: 95.7%	CC: 80.0% Chromo: 87.5% NBI: 87.5%	CC: 79.1% Chromo: 92.7% NBI: 92.7%
Chiu et al[83]	2007	Prospective; polyp analysis	133	Dense vascular network or brown vascular pattern	CC: 62.1%–65.2% Chromo: 78.7%–85.1% NBI: 82.3%–86.5%	CC: 74.4%–85.4% Chromo: 79.5%–84.6% NBI: 59.0%–82.7%	CC: 67.2%–68.3% Chromo: 78.9%–85.0% NBI: 80.6%–82.4%
East et al[73]	2007	Prospective comparative study (all HD colonoscopes)	20	Kudo classification and vascular pattern	Chromo: 64% NBI pit pattern: 77% NBI vessel intensity: 77%	Chromo: 90% NBI pit pattern: 60% NBI vessel intensity: 50%	Chromo: 72% NBI pit pattern: 72% NBI vessel intensity: 69%
Tischendorf et al[76]	2007	Randomized to magnifying NBI vs magnifying chromo	99	Kudo classification and vascular pattern	Pit pattern: MConv: 63.4% MChromo: 91.7% NBI: 90.5% Vessel pattern: MConv: 47.2% Chromo: 66.7% NBI: 93.7%	Pit pattern: MConv: 51.9% MChromo: 90.0% NBI: 89.2% Vessel pattern: MConv: 97.4% Chromo: 95.0% NBI: 89.2%	Pit pattern: MConv: 59.0% MChromo: 91.0% NBI: 90.0% Vessel pattern: MConv: 66.5% Chromo: 78.0% NBI: 92.0%
Rastogi et al[75]	2009	Prospective comparative study	100	Surface pattern/vascular pattern	HDWL: 38% NBI: 96%	HDWL: 97% NBI: 89%	HDWL: 61% NBI: 93%

Abbreviations: CC, conventional colonoscopy; HDWL, high-definition white light; MChromo, magnifying chromoendoscopy; MConv, magnifying conventional colonoscopy; NBI, narrow band imaging.

high-definition white light, followed by NBI without magnification and chromoendoscopy.[84] In 130 subjects, 363 polyps less than 10 mm were detected, of which 278 polyps had both an optical and histopathological diagnosis. Histology confirmed that 198 of these polyps were adenomas and 80 were non-neoplastic lesions (of which 62 were hyperplastic). Optical diagnosis accurately characterized 186 of 198 polyps as adenomas (sensitivity 0.94; 95% CI 0.90–0.97) and 55 of 62 polyps as hyperplastic (specificity 0.89; 0.78–0.95), with an overall accuracy of 241 of 260 (0.93; 0.89–0.96) for polyp characterization. In 82 of 130 subjects, physicians could give a surveillance interval to the subject immediately after colonoscopy, with concordant intervals in 98% of subjects using British guidelines after formal histopathology.

The researchers concluded that in vivo optical diagnosis could be used for polyps less than 10 mm to assess polyp histopathology and future surveillance intervals. Dispensing with formal histopathology for most small polyps found at colonoscopy could save money, time, and potentially patient compliance.

Douglas Rex proposed that an application of confidence levels to optical diagnoses of adenomatous polyps versus hyperplastic histology could further boost performance to greater than 90% for NBI predictions of adenomas and hyperplastic polyps. In his study, 92% of all high-confidence adenomatous polyps were correct and 95% of all high-confidence hyperplastic polyps were correct.[85] However, Kuiper and colleagues caution practitioners that for safe clinical use, the sensitivity of NBI should approach 100% before we can completely rely on optical diagnoses because leaving adenomas in situ would be harmful to patients.[86] Future studies should assess NBI sensitivity with diminutive adenomas and assess interobserver variability of NBI determinations before this technology can be used mainstream.

Data on interobserver agreement for NBI assessment varies. In 32 polyps by 2 observers, East and colleagues[73] determined a κ value of 0.48 for kudo pit pattern and 0.64 for vascular pattern intensity. Su and colleagues[74] reported a κ value of 1.0 by 2 assessors who scored for brownish vascular network among 110 colorectal polyps. Tischendorf and colleagues[76] also stated perfect agreement for NBI by 2 observers of 200 polyps based on mucosal and vascular patterns.

FICE

Other digital imaging technologies exist to enhance mucosal contrast. Computed virtual chromoscopy with the Fujinon Intelligent Color Enhancement system is a new imaging technique that can narrow the bandwidth of light components, like NBI, to enhance mucosal contrast. FICE relies on a computed spectral estimation technology that processes reflected photons to recreate a virtual image at different wavelengths. It has up to 10 setting functions that allow for different imaging settings during the examination.

To date, 2 prospective studies have examined the utility of FICE in improving adenoma detection rates. In a study by Pohl and colleagues,[87] 871 subjects were randomized to FICE mode colonoscopy versus standard colonoscopy with targeted indigo carmine chromoscopy in consecutive subjects having screening colonoscopies. Final enrollment included 764 subjects and there was no significant difference in number of adenomas detected between the FICE group and the chromoendoscopy group (271 vs 236, p = ns) and there was no significant difference in number of subjects with greater than or equal to 1 adenoma between the FICE and chromoendoscopy group (35.6% vs 35.4%). For the subgroup of flat lesions, there was even a trend toward poorer detection with FICE. However, FICE was able to more accurately distinguish between non-neoplastic and neoplastic lesions with a sensitivity of 92.7% compared with chromoendoscopy (90.4%). However, this was not statistically significant.

A recent prospective trial of 359 average-risk subjects for colon cancer randomized to tandem colonoscopy with either FICE colonoscopy first or standard white light, high-resolution colonoscopy first revealed once again that adenoma detection rates were not significantly improved with FICE.[85] The adenoma detection rates were high in both groups (FICE: 0.64 vs WL: 0.55 per subject; $P = .65$) and may have masked the diagnostic benefit of FICE. However, technically, the investigators state that FICE had insufficient brightness to ensure good visualization of the colonic mucosa. Furthermore, according to the investigators, intestinal fluid impedes visualization with FICE more than WLE. The high magnification mode is useful for detailed inspection of targeted areas but was considered technically challenging in this study.

I-SCAN

Another postprocessing light-filter technology is called i-scan by Pentax. This imaging platform relies on a variety of filters with more pixels in the CCD to refine the digital image.[88,89] There are several modes that can be used to evaluate the mucosa, including surface enhancement (SE)-mode for surface analysis, v-mode for vessel characterization, and p-mode for pattern characterization. The surface-enhancement mode is meant to be used on withdrawal and the p and v modes are used to further assess histology and differentiate between hyperplastic and adenomatous lesions (see **Fig. 3**).

One prospective study examined the role of i-scan in detecting small lesions less than 5 mm compared with HD colonoscopy alone or HD colonoscopy with methylene blue chromoendoscopy. The order of the imaging modalities were randomized but always ended in chromoendoscopy and the last 30 cm were inspected with this technology. In 69 subjects, i-scan increased lesion detection from 176 with HD to 335 with HD and i-scan ($P<.001$). With the addition of chromoendoscopy, 646 lesions were detected ($P<.001$), but chromoendoscopy did not increase the detection rate of neoplasia beyond that which was found with i-scan (HD [4] vs i-scan[11] vs chromoendoscopy [11]). However, the sensitivity of 82% in determining adenomatous lesions may still be too low to provide a definitive optical diagnosis without histologic confirmation[90] Larger studies will need to confirm these findings. I-scan may be able to help detect smaller lesions as efficiently as chromoendoscopy, but with decreased procedural time.

SUMMARY

New high-resolution colonoscopes and filter technologies are allowing us to visualize more lesions and better characterize lesions within the GI tract. In light of recent findings that flat and serrated lesions are more likely to contain invasive cancer and that even small lesions (5–10 mm) may contain advanced histology, detecting these lesions earlier with improved optical technologies may help decrease the rate of interval cancers after colonoscopy. With the limited accuracy of white-light colonoscopy (59%–84%) in distinguishing non-neoplastic lesions from neoplastic lesions, these new technologies can help us improve our abilities to risk stratify patients and determine more precise surveillance intervals. Furthermore, we may be able to see significant cost savings if optical diagnoses can accurately detect neoplastic lesions, allowing us to determine long-term surveillance intervals more efficiently and reduce the number of biopsies evaluated by pathology.[75,76,81,84]

Parallel efforts should focus on understanding the natural history of these difficult to visualize, flat and diminutive lesions. The role of these new technologies in clinical practice will depend on the significance of these lesions. Furthermore, quality improvement measures should continue as skilled operator performance continues to play a significant role in improving adenoma detection rates.[91] Future studies should also attempt to define learning curves for these new technologies and determine which patient populations would benefit most from a given technology as they become incorporated into everyday clinical practice.

REFERENCES

1. Singh H, Turner D, Xue L, et al. Risk of developing colorectal cancer following a negative colonoscopy examination: evidence for a 10-year interval between colonoscopies. JAMA 2006;295:2366–73.
2. Schatzkin A, Lanza E, Corle D, et al. The polyp prevention trial study group. Lack of effect of a low-fat, high-fiber diet on the recurrence of colorectal adenomas. N Engl J Med 2000;342:1149–55.
3. Robertson DJ, Greenberg ER, Beach M, et al. Colorectal cancer in patients under close colonoscopic surveillance. Gastroenterology 2005;129:34–41.
4. Alberts D, Martinez M, Roe D, et al. The phoenix colon cancer prevention physicians' network. Lack of effect of a high-fiber cereal supplement on the recurrence of colorectal adenomas. N Engl J Med 2000;342:1156–62.
5. Winawer SJ, Zauber AG, Ho MN, et al. Prevention of colorectal cancer by colonoscopic polypectomy. The national polyp study workgroup. N Engl J Med 1993; 329:1977–81.
6. Citarda F, Tomaselli G, Capocaccia R, et al. Efficacy in standard clinical practice of colonoscopic polypectomy in reducing colorectal cancer incidence. Gut 2001; 48:812–5.
7. Soetikno RM, Kaltenbach T, Rouse RV, et al. Prevalence of nonpolypoid (Flat and Depressed) colorectal neoplasms in asymptomatic and symptomatic adults. JAMA 2008;299(9):1027–35.
8. Van Rijn JC, Reitsma JB, Stoker J, et al. Polyp miss rate determined by tandem colonoscopy: a systematic review. Am J Gastroenterol 2006;101:343–50.
9. Rex D, Helbig C. High yields of small and flat adenomas with high definition colonoscopes using either white light or narrow band imaging. Gastroenterology 2007;133:42–7.
10. East JE, Stavrindis M, Thomas-Gibson S, et al. A Comparative study of standard vs. high definition colonoscopy for adenoma and hyperplastic polyp detection with optimized withdrawal technique. Aliment Pharmacol Ther 2008;28:768–76.
11. Pellise M, Fernandez-Esparrach G, Cardenas A, et al. Impact of wide-angle, high-definition endoscopy in the diagnosis of colorectal neoplasia: a randomized controlled trial. Gastroenterology 2008;135(4):1062–8.
12. Tribonias G, Theodoropoulou A, Konstantinidis K, et al. Comparison of standard versus high-definition, wide-angle colonoscopy for polyp detection: a randomized controlled trial. Colorectal Dis 2010;12:e260–6.
13. Burke CA, Choure AG, Sanaka MR, et al. A Comparison of high-definition versus conventional colonoscopes for polyp detection. Dig Dis Sci 2010;55:1716–20.
14. Buchner AM, Shahid MW, Kechman MG, et al. High definition colonoscopy detects colorectal polyps at a higher rate than standard white light colonoscopy. Clin Gastroenterol Hepatol 2010;8(4):364–70.
15. Hoffman A, Sar F, Goetz M, et al. High definition colonoscopy combined with i-scan is superior in the detection of colorectal neoplasias compared to standard video colonoscopy – a prospective randomized controlled trial. Endoscopy 2010; 42:827–33.
16. Read TE, Read JD, Butterly LF. Importance of adenomas 5 mm or less in diameter that are detected by sigmoidoscopy. N Engl J Med 1997;336:8–12.

17. Church JM. Clinical significance of small colorectal polyps. Dis Colon Rectum 2004;47:481–5.
18. Butterly LF, Chase MP, Pohl H, et al. Prevalence of clinically important histology in small adenomas. Clin Gastroenterol Hepatol 2006;4:343–8.
19. Olliver JR, Wild CP, Sahay P, et al. Chromoendoscopy with methylene blue and associated DNA damage in Barrett's oesophagus. Lancet 2003;362:373–4.
20. Davies J, Burke D, Olliver JR, et al. Methylene blue but not indigo carmine causes DNA damage to colonocytes in vitro and in vivo at concentrations used in clinical chromoendoscopy. Gut 2007;56:155–6.
21. Dinis-Ribeiro M, Moreira-Dias L. There is no clinical evidence of consequences after methylene blue chromoendoscopy. Gastrointest Endosc 2008; 67:1209.
22. Brown SR, Baraza W, Hurlstone DP. Chromoscopy versus conventional endoscopy for the detection of polyps in the colon and rectum. Cochrane Database Syst Rev 2007;4:CD006439.
23. Brooker JC, Saunders BP, Shah SG, et al. Total colonic dye-spray increases the detection of diminutive adenomas during routine colonoscopy; a randomized controlled trial. Gastrointest Endosc 2002;56:333–8.
24. Le Rhun M, Coron E, Parlier D, et al. High resolution colonoscopy with chromoscopy versus standard colonoscopy for the detection of colonic neoplasia: a randomized study. Clin Gastroenterol Hepatol 2006;4:349–54.
25. Hurlstone DP, Cross SS, Slater R, et al. Detecting diminutive colorectal lesions at colonoscopy: a randomized controlled trial of pan-colonic versus targeted chromoendoscopy. Gut 2004;53:376.
26. Lapalus MG, Helbert T, Napoleon B, et al. Does chromoendoscopy with structure enhancement improve the colonoscopic adenoma detection rate? Endoscopy 2006;38(5):444–8.
27. Rembacken BJ, Fujii T, Cairns A, et al. Flat and depressed colonic neoplasms: a prospective study of 1000 colonoscopies in the UK. Lancet 2000;355: 1211–4.
28. Lee JH, Kim JW, Cho YK, et al. Detection of colorectal adenomas by routine chromoendoscopy with indigo carmine. Am J Gastroenterol 2003;98:1284–8.
29. Stoffel EM, Turgeon DK, Stockwell DH, et al. Chromoendoscopy detects more adenomas than colonoscopy using intensive inspection without dye spraying. Cancer Prev Res 2008;1(7):507–13.
30. Park SY, Lee SK, Kim BC, et al. Efficacy of chromoendoscopy with indigocarmine for the detection of ascending colon and cecum lesions. Scand J Gastroenterol 2008;43:878–85.
31. Kudo S, Hirota S, Nakajima T, et al. Colorectal tumors and pit pattern. J Clin Pathol 1994;47:880–5.
32. Davila R. Chromoendoscopy. Gastrointest Endosc Clin N Am 2009;19:193–208.
33. Fu KI, Sano Y, Kato S, et al. Chromoendoscopy using indigo carmine dye spraying with magnifying observation is the most reliable method for differential diagnosis between non-neoplastic and neoplastic colorectal lesions: a prospective study. Endoscopy 2004;36:1089–93.
34. Kato S, Fukii T, Koba I, et al. Assessment of colorectal lesions using magnifying colonoscopy and mucosal dye spraying; can significant lesions be distinguished? Endoscopy 2001;33:306–10.
35. Su MY, Ho YP, Chen PC, et al. Magnifying endoscopy with indigo carmine contrast for differential diagnosis of neoplastic and nonneoplastic colonic polyps. Dig Dis Sci 2004;49:1123–7.

36. Axelrad A, Fleischer DE, Geller AJ, et al. High-resolution chromoendoscopy for the diagnosis of diminutive colon polyps: implications for colon cancer screening. Gastroenterology 1996;110:1253–8.

37. Togashi K, Konishi F, Ishizuka T, et al. Efficacy of magnifying endoscopy in the differential diagnosis of neoplastic and non-neoplastic polyps of the large bowel. Dis Colon Rectum 1999;42:1602–8.

38. Tung SY, Wu CS, Su MY. Magnifying colonoscopy in differentiating neoplastic from nonneoplastic colorectal lesions. Am J Gastroenterol 2001;96:2628–32.

39. Eisen GM, Kim CY, Fleischer DE, et al. High-resolution chromoendoscopy for classifying colonic polyps: a multicenter study. Gastrointest Endosc 2002;55:687–94.

40. Konishi K, Kaneko K, Kurahashi T, et al. A comparison of magnifying and non-magnifying colonoscopy for diagnosis of colorectal polyps: a prospective study. Gastrointest Endosc 2003;57:48–53.

41. Hurlstone DP, Cross SS, Adam I, et al. Efficacy of high magnification chromoscopic colonoscopy for the diagnosis of neoplasia in flat and depressed lesions of the colorectum: a prospective analysis. Gut 2004;53:284–90.

42. Huang Q, Fukami N. Interobserver and intra-observer consistency in the endoscopic assessment of colonic pit pattern. Gastrointest Endosc 2004;60(4):520–6.

43. Apel D, Jakobs R, Schilling D, et al. Accuracy of high-resolution chromoendoscopy in prediction of histologic findings in diminutive lesions of the rectosigmoid. Gastrointest Endosc 2006;63:824–8.

44. De Francisco J, Grady WM. Diagnosis and management of hereditary non-polyposis colon cancer. Gastrointest Endosc 2003;58:390–408.

45. Vasen H, Taal BG, Nagengast FM. Hereditary nonpolyposis colorectal cancer: result of long-term surveillance in 50 families. Eur J Cancer 1995;31A:1145–8.

46. Hurlstone DP, Karajeh M, Cross SS, et al. The role of high-magnification-chromoscopic colonoscopy in hereditary nonpolyposis colorectal cancer screening: a prospective "back-to-back" endoscopic study. Am J Gastroenterol 2005;100: 2167–73.

47. Lecomte T, Cellier C, Meatchi T, et al. Chromoendoscopic colonoscopy for detecting preneoplastic lesions in hereditary nonpolyposis colorectal cancer syndrome. Clin Gastroenterol Hepatol 2005;3(9):897–902.

48. Stoffel E, Turgeon DK, Stockwell DH. Missed adenomas during colonoscopic surveillance in individuals with lynch syndrome. Cancer Prev Res 2008;1:470–5.

49. Shelton AA, Lehman RE, Schrock TR, et al. Retrospective review of colorectal cancer in ulcerative colitis at a tertiary center. Arch Surg 1996;131:806–10.

50. Eaden JA, Abrams KR, Mayberry JF. The risk of colorectal cancer in ulcerative colitis: a meta-analysis. Gut 2001;48:526–35.

51. Rutter MD, Saunders BP, Wilkinson KH, et al. Thirty-year analysis of a colonoscopic surveillance program from neoplasia in ulcerative colitis. Gastro 2006;130:1030–8.

52. Rutter MD. Are dysplasia and colorectal cancer endoscopically visible in patients with ulcerative colitis? Gastrointest Endosc 2008;67:1009–10.

53. Sada M, Igarashi M, Yoshizawa S, et al. Dye spraying and magnifying endoscopy for dysplasia and cancer surveillance in ulcerative colitis. Dis Colon Rectum 2004;47:1816–23.

54. Kiesslich R, Fritsch J, Holtmann M, et al. Methylene blue-aided chromoendoscopy for the detection of intraepithelial neoplasia and colon cancer in ulcerative colitis. Gastroenterology 2003;124:880–8.

55. Kiesslich R, Goetz M, Lammersdorf K, et al. Chromoscopy-guided endomicroscopy increases the diagnostic yield of intraepithelial neoplasia in ulcerative colitis. Gastroenterology 2007;132:874–82.

56. Hurlstone DP, Sanders DS, Lobo AJ, et al. Indigo carmine-assisted high-magnification chromoscopic colonoscopy for the detection and characterisation of intraepithelial neoplasia in UC: a prospective evaluation. Endoscopy 2005;37: 1186–92.
57. Rutter MD, Saunders BP, Schofield G, et al. Pancolonic indigo carmine dye spraying for the detection of dysplasia in ulcerative colitis. Gut 2004;53: 256–60.
58. Marion JF, Waye JD, Present DH. Chromoendoscopy-targeted biopsies are superior to standard colonoscopic surveillance for detecting dysplasia in inflammatory bowel disease patients: a prospective endoscopic trial. Am J Gastroenterol 2008; 103:2342–9.
59. Matsumoto T, Nakamura S, Jo Y, et al. Chromoscopy might improve diagnostic accuracy in cancer surveillance for ulcerative colitis. Am J Gastroenterol 2003; 98:1827–33.
60. Farraye FA, Odze RD, Eaden J, et al. AGA Institute Medical Position Panel on Diagnosis and Management of Colorectal Neoplasia in Inflammatory Bowel Disease. AGA medical position statement on the diagnosis and management of colorectal neoplasia in inflammatory bowel disease. Gastroenterology 2010;138(2):738–45.
61. Biancone L, Michetti P, Travis S, et al. European evidence-based consensus on the management of ulcerative colitis: special situations. J Crohns Colitis 2008; 2:63–92.
62. Kaltenbach T, Friedland S, Soetikno R. A randomized tandem colonoscopy trial of narrow band imaging versus white light examination to compare neoplasia miss rates. Gut 2008;57:1406–12.
63. Adler A, Aschenbeck J, Yenerim T, et al. Narrow-band versus white-light high definition television endoscopic imaging for screening colonoscopy: a prospective randomized trial 2009;136(2):410–6.
64. Adler A, Pohl H, Papnikolaou S, et al. A prospective randomized study on narrow-band imaging versus conventional colonoscopy for adenoma detection: does narrow-band imaging induce a learning effect? Gut 2008;57:59–64.
65. Paggi S, Radaelli F, Amato A, et al. The impact of narrow band imaging in screening colonoscopy: A randomized controlled trial. Clin Gastroenterol Hepatol 2009;7:1049–164.
66. Inoue T, Mirano M, Murano N, et al. Comparative study of conventional colonoscopy and pan-colonic narrow band imaging system in the detection of neoplastic colonic polyps: a randomized control trial. J Gastroenterol 2008;43:45–50.
67. East JF, Suzuki N, Stavrinidis M. Narrow band imaging for colonoscopic surveillance in hereditary non-polyposis colorectal cancer. Gut 2008;57:65–70.
68. Huneburg R, Lammert F, Rabe C, et al. Chromocolonoscopy detects more adenomas than white light colonoscopy or narrow band imaging colonoscopy in hereditary nonpolyposis colorectal cancer screening. Endoscopy 2009;41: 316–22.
69. Dekker E, van den Broek FJC, Hardwich JC, et al. Narrow-band imaging compared with conventional colonoscopy for the detection of dysplasia in patients with longstanding ulcerative colitis. Endoscopy 2007;39:216–21.
70. Matsumoto T, Kudo T, Jo Y, et al. Magnifying colonoscopy with narrow band imaging system for the diagnosis of dysplasia in ulcerative colitis: a pilot study. Gastrointest Endosc 2007;66:957–65.
71. van den Broek FJ, Fockens P, van Eeden S, et al. Endoscopic tri-modal imaging for surveillance in ulcerative colitis: randomized comparison of high resolution endoscopy and autofluorescence imaging for neoplasia detection;

and evaluation of narrow band imaging for classification of lesions. Gut 2008; 57:1083–9.

72. East JE, Saunders BP. Narrow band imaging at colonoscopy: seeing through a glass darkly or the light of a new dawn? Expert Rev Gastroenterol Hepatol 2008;2:1–4.

73. East JE, Suzuki N, Saunders BP. Comparison of magnified pit pattern interpretation with narrow band imaging versus chromoendoscopy for diminutive colonic polyps: a pilot study. Gastrointest Endosc 2007;66:310–6.

74. Su MY, Hsu CM, Ho YP, et al. Comparative study of conventional colonoscopy, chromoendoscopy, and narrow-band imaging systems in differential diagnosis of neoplastic and nonneoplastic colonic polyps. Am J Gastroenterol 2006;101: 2711–6.

75. Rastogi A, Keighley J, Singh V, et al. High Accuracy of Narrow Band Imaging without Magnification for the Real Time Characterization of Polyp Histology and Its Comparison with White Light Colonoscopy: A Prospective Study. Am J Gastro 2009;104:2422–30.

76. Tischendorf JJ, Wasmuth HE, Koch A, et al. Value of magnifying chromoendoscopy and narrow band imaging (NBI) in classifying colorectal polyps: a prospective controlled study. Endoscopy 2007;39:1092–6.

77. Katagiri A, Fu KI, Sano Y, et al. Narrow band imaging with magnifying colonoscopy as a diagnostic tool for predicting the histology of early colorectal neoplasia. Aliment Pharmacol Ther 2008;27:1269–74.

78. Hirata M, Tanaka S, Oka S, et al. Magnifying endoscopy with narrow band imaging for diagnosis of colorectal tumors. Gastrointest Endosc 2007;65: 988–95.

79. Hirata M, Tanaka S, Oka S, et al. Evaluation of microvessels in colorectal tumors by narrow band imaging magnification. Gastrointest Endosc 2007;66: 945–52.

80. Sikka S, Ringold DA, Jonnalagadda S, et al. Comparison of white light and narrow band high definition images in predicting colon polyp histology, using standard colonoscopies without optical magnification. Endoscopy 2008;40:818–22.

81. Machida H, Sano Y, Hamamoto Y, et al. Narrow-band imaging in the diagnosis of colorectal mucosal lesions: a pilot study. Endoscopy 2004;36:1094–8.

82. van den Broek FJ, Reitsma JB, Curvers WL, et al. Systematic review of narrow-band imaging for the detection and differentiation of neoplastic and nonneoplastic lesions. Gastrointest Endosc 2009;69:124–35.

83. Chiu HM, Chang CY, Chen CC, et al. A prospective comparative study of narrow-band imaging, chromoendoscopy, and conventional colonoscopy in the diagnosis of colorectal neoplasia. Gut 2007;56:373–9.

84. Ignjatovic A, East JE, Suzuki N, et al. Optical diagnosis of small colorectal polyps at routine colonoscopy (detect inspect characterise resect and discard; DISCARD trial): a prospective study. Lancet Oncol 2009;10:1171–8.

85. Rex D. Narrow-Band Imaging Without Optical Magnification for Histologic Analysis of Colorectal Polyps 2009. Gastroenterology 2009;136:1174–81.

86. Kuiper T, Dekker E. NBI detection and differentiation of colonic lesions. Nature Review Gastroenterology and Hepatology 2010;7:128–30.

87. Pohl J, Lotterer E, Balzer C, et al. Computed virtual chromoendoscopy versus standard colonoscopy with targeted indigo carmine chromoscopy: a randomized mulicentre trial. Gut 2009;58:73–8.

88. Atkinson M, Chak A. I-scan: chromoendoscopy without the hassle? Dig Liver Dis 2010;42:18–9.

89. Kodashima S, Fujishoro M. Novel image-enhanced endoscopy with i-scan technology. World J Gastroenterol 2010;16:1043–9.
90. Hoffman A, Kagel C, Goetz M, et al. Recognition and characterization of small colonic neoplasia with high-definition colonoscopy using i-scan is as precise as chromoendoscopy. Dig Liver Dis 2010;42:45–50.
91. Rex DK, Cutler CS, Lemmet GT, et al. Colonoscopic withdrawal technique is associated with adenoma miss rates. Gastrointest Endosc 2000;51:33–6.

Wide View and Retroview During Colonoscopy

Jerome D. Waye, MD

KEYWORDS

- Wide-angle colonoscope • Retroview in the colon
- Third-eye retroscope • Retroflexion • New instrument

Colonoscopy has long been considered the gold standard for evaluation of the colon, as not only can it locate and find lesions throughout the large intestine, but therapy is also possible during the procedure. Unfortunately, time has shown that colonoscopy may be a flawed gold standard, as lesions may be missed and carcinomas may not be prevented. In an editorial, Dr David Lieberman[1] stated that "the data on colonoscopy accuracy is a humble reminder of the limitations of colonoscopy." Despite the known diagnostic accuracy of colonoscopy, this examination may miss some colonic lesions.

Colonoscopy became popular soon after it was introduced because it was a considerably better tool than barium for colonic evaluation. However, early in the infancy of this combined diagnostic and therapeutic procedure, investigators questioned the accuracy of this gold standard. It was decided that the best way to test the accuracy of colonoscopy was to have a procedure performed and immediately afterward have a repeat examination by the same or a different endoscopist. Thus the patient would serve as his or her own control and permit the discovery of any lesions missed by the first examiner.

The concept of "tandem colonoscopy" is best suited for evaluation of a discrete lesion such as a polyp because this is a quantifiable object with a defined size, shape, and location in the colon. If seen and removed, biopsied, or photographed, there is no mistake that it is present. During these investigations, the first examiner removes all polyps that are encountered so that all polyps seen by the second endoscopist will represent overlooked lesions. One drawback to tandem colonoscopy is that the interventionists are totally aware that this study is under way and will pay special attention to the intraluminal pathology so as not to miss lesions. Despite the heightened awareness by virtue of participating in a tandem colonoscopy experiment, the 3 trials that specifically evaluated the possible "miss" rate of polyps in the large bowel revealed

Disclosures: none.
Mount Sinai Hospital, World Endoscopy Organization (OMED), Mount Sinai Medical Center, 650 Park Avenue, New York, NY 10065, USA
E-mail address: Jdwaye@aol.com

Gastroenterol Clin N Am 39 (2010) 883–900
doi:10.1016/j.gtc.2010.08.033
0889-8553/10/$ – see front matter © 2010 Elsevier Inc. All rights reserved.

gastro.theclinics.com

strikingly large numbers of polyps overlooked by the first examiner using standard colonoscopic equipment.

The first report of back-to-back colonoscopies on the same day and immediately following each other was in 1991.[2] The next report of tandem colonoscopy appeared 6 years later,[3] and the most recent was in 2008.[4] The overall miss rates for adenomas in the earlier studies[2,3] were 15% to 24%. The large multicenter European study[4] found that the miss rate for all polyps was 28%, for hyperplastic polyps 31%, and for adenomas 21%. However, the miss rate for all polyps equal to or larger than 5 mm was 12% and for adenomas 9%. Among the 14 polyps and 6 adenomas larger than 5 mm missed during the first examination, 5 polyps and 1 adenoma were sessile, and 9 polyps and 5 adenomas were flat. In all, 37 adenomas were overlooked in 286 patients with the median size being 3 mm; however, the range of missed lesions was from 1 to 18 mm. In this European study, 3 advanced adenomas were missed with a size from 15 to 18 mm. The investigators reported that there was a 27% rate of missed adenomas for lesions smaller than 5 mm in diameter, and the miss rate for lesions greater than 5 mm in diameter was 9%. In a previous study of 183 patients having tandem colonoscopy, Rex and colleagues[3] reported a 27% miss rate for polyps smaller than 6 mm in diameter and only 6% for polyps larger than 9 mm. There was no significant difference between in the miss rate of polyps in the right colon (27%) and the left colon (21%). Although a substantial percentage (24%) of adenomas was missed, there was an inverse ratio between the miss rate and the size of the adenoma. In the summary of the report, Rex and colleagues recommended that technology be developed that may overcome the technical limitations of colonoscopy.

Another way of evaluating whether polyps were missed on an initial colonoscopic examination is to repeat the colonoscopy at an interval time, not on the same day as the original procedure. In a retrospective analysis[5] of more than 15,000 colonoscopies, the polyp miss rate was evaluated by comparing findings on repeat colonoscopic examinations at 4 and 12 months after the initial colonoscopic examination. The calculated miss rate for all polyps was 17% and for neoplastic polyps 12%. Retrospective studies such as this are not as elegant as tandem examinations, but the findings are similar: polyps are missed during the initial colonoscopy.

The problem with missed colonoscopic neoplasms is primarily due to their location, being on the proximal aspect of folds; this means that the technique of the examination is critically important in the discovery of colon polyps. It has been shown that not all missed lesions are "hidden" because flat neoplasms can elude detection by the casual or untrained observer,[6] even when they are in the field of view of the straightforward viewing standard colonoscope. Pickhardt and colleagues[7] did a computed tomographic colonography (CTC) evaluation of more than 1200 persons who had same-day CTC and colonoscopy. With segmental unblinding during a colonoscopic examination that followed the CTC, 10% of polyps were found only after they were originally missed by colonoscopy but detected on the original CTC. Of the missed neoplasms found on the second-look colonoscopy after segmental unblinding, 17 were tubular adenomas, 3 were tubulovillous adenomas, and 1 was a small adenocarcinoma (size range 6–17 mm). The majority of these neoplasms were located on the edge or on the proximal aspect of a fold.[7] A more recent article from London[8] on CTC simulation reconstructions using a 90° imaging field of view corroborated a previous report[9] which showed that 23.4% of the colonic surface is not visualized by direct straight end-on examinations. The report by East and colleagues[8] repeated the type of scan by Pickhardt and colleagues[9] but with simulated varying fields of view of 90°, 120°, 140°, and 170° to match the angle of view of some colonoscopes. In addition, a simulated retrograde view was obtained with a 135° field of view, equivalent to retrograde viewing by the third-eye retroscope (TER). In this study,[8] the percentage of visualized colonic surface increased with each increasing angle of view increment. The total number of missed areas was approximately the same for fields of view of 90° to 140°, but decreased when the field of view was 170°. Approximately only 85% of the colonic surface would be visualized using a 140° angle of view, and this increased so that more of the surface would be seen when the examination was repeated using a 170° angle of view comparable to the Olympus 180 series colonoscopes (Olympus Medical Instruments, Tokyo, Japan). The simulated addition of a retrograde viewing auxiliary imaging device led to an almost complete surface visualization, with a tenfold decrease in the area that was missed compared with that obtained using a wide-angle colonoscope with a 170° angle of view. With the simulation of optical colonoscopy by CTC software, using the commonly available 140° angle of view of most colono-scopes, approximately 13% of the colonic surface is unseen. Simulation of a colono-scope with a 170° field of view resulted in an almost 6% reduction in percentage of surface missed. The marked additional mucosal visualization seen in the simulation models with a combination of 140° forward and a 135° reverse view (such as that provided by the TER) may actually be preferred to recently developed optics providing a 360° view (Aer-O-Scope),[10] which has a substantial "fish eye effect." In this simula-tion model, there does not seem to be any additional benefit to using a colonoscope with 170° angle of view instead of a 140° instrument when associated with the addi-tional advantage of the TER.

Barthel,[11] in an editorial in *Gastrointestinal Endoscopy*, mentions that to attempt an increase in the finding of adenomas, there have been several articles written on the use of a wide-angle lens on a colonoscope. At present, most colonoscopes have a 140° angle of view, but only one manufacturer has a standard production model colono-scope with a 170° angle of view (Olympus Medical Endoscope, Tokyo, Japan) (**Figs. 1** and **2**). An evaluation of a 15-mm diameter colonoscope with a 210° angle of view,[12] in which the lens projects from the endoscope tip permitting an ultrawide angle of view, has been performed. With this instrument, the viewing angle could be converted to 160° for close inspection of the mucosal surface. This study included 50 patients randomized to the ultrawide-angle colonoscope compared with a standard colonoscope with a 140° angle of view. There was no difference between the 2 types of colonoscopes in the detection of adenomas, but the miss rate for polyps was some-what lower with the ultrawide-angle colonoscope. It is interesting that of two exam-iners, one found no difference in adenoma detection between the 2 types of

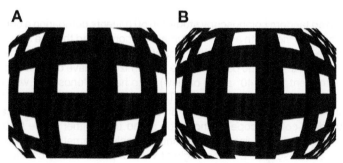

Fig. 1. Identical flat grids showing the width of view obtained by (*A*) a standard colono-scope with a 140° angle of view (Olympus CF-Q160AL; Olympus Instrument Company, Tokyo, Japan) and (*B*) an instrument with a 170° angle of view (Olympus CF-Q180AL).

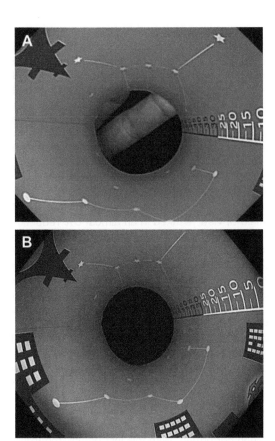

Fig. 2. Identical cones to show the image obtained by colonoscopes with differing angles of view, held at the same distance from the tip of the lens of (*A*) a standard colonoscope (140° angle of view) and (*B*) a wide-angle colonoscope (170° angle of view).

colonoscopes, but the second examiner missed more polyps with the ultrawide-angle colonoscope than when using a colonoscope with a 140° angle of view. The investigators concluded that the principal deficit of the extremely wide-angle colonoscope was that the resolution was significantly reduced when compared with standard colonoscopes.

A randomized tandem colonoscopy study[13] in 50 patients comparing a colonoscope with a 170° angle of view with a 140° instrument demonstrated that the miss rate for all polyps with the wide-angle colonoscope was similar to the miss rate with the standard colonoscope. In this study, 50 patients were randomized to have colonoscopy with the standard instrument first (140° angle of view) or to have colonoscopy with the wide-angle instrument as the first examination. The miss rate for all polyps with the wide-angle colonoscope was not statistically different from the miss rate for all polyps with the standard colonoscope. It should be noted that neither of the tested instruments were high-definition instruments, and the only parameter that was different between the 2 endoscopes was the angle of view of the lens. The conclusion of the investigators was that "in comparison with other innovations for reducing polyp miss rates during colonoscopy ... wide angle colonoscopy may be the least effective strategy." A similar conclusion was reached by a group from Spain[14] who randomized, in a one-to-one ratio, 620 patients into those having colonoscopy with a wide-angle high-definition instrument versus procedures using a standard colonoscope. This study showed no significant difference in the number of adenomas detected by either instrument. A study[15] with 8 colonoscopists at 2 institutions randomized 710 patients using a standard (140° angle of view) colonoscope and a 170° wide-angle instrument. Neither instrument had a high-definition component. The primary end point of this study was to see if there was a reduction in withdrawal time using the wide-angle instrument as compared with the standard colonoscope. The mean insertion time for the 2 instruments was similar, at approximately 5 minutes, but overall the mean withdrawal time was shorter with the wide-angle colonoscope than with the standard colonoscope (4.9 vs 5.4 minutes); however, the shorter withdrawal time was only statistically significant for 3 of the 8 endoscopists. In this study, the proportion of patients with at least one adenoma was significantly higher for the standard instrument than for the wide-angle colonoscope. However, there was no difference in the mean number of adenomas detected with either instrument. The conclusion was that although there was a 30-second reduction in mean withdrawal time using wide-angle instruments, the benefits of the wide-angle colonoscope "appeared minimal on close inspection."

In contrast to the majority of reports, a nonrandomized study from Prague[16] compared wide-angle high-definition colonoscopy with standard-angle (140°) instruments with and without high definition. A total of 507 patients were involved in the study, which showed that the wide-angle high-definition instrument detected more adenomas, flat adenomas, and adenomas with advanced histology as compared with both instruments with a 140° angle of view. The instruments were not randomly assigned in this study, but the mean rate of adenomas and flat adenomas found per patient was significantly higher in the wide-angle high-definition colonoscopic group compared with the other groups, and in the right colon was almost double that found with the standard-angle colonoscopes. The currently available 170° wide-angle instrument also has a high-definition component. The question arises as to whether the high-definition component increases the ability of the examiner to find more polyps and adenomas than can be found with the wide-angle component alone.

A retrospective report from the Cleveland Clinic[17] compared endoscopic findings in more than 400 individuals who underwent examination with a wide-angle high-definition colonoscope and compared them with a group who had conventional colonoscopy (non–high definition) with a 140° angle of view that were matched for gender, age, and indication for colonoscopy. This study was not randomized, and polyps were detected in 39.9% of the subjects in the high-definition/wide-angle group and in 36.9% of those in the conventional colonoscopy group. The investigators concluded that wide-angle high-definition colonoscopy afforded no increase in the detection of polyps or adenomas over conventional colonoscopy with 140° angle of view, and that the improved resolution and wider angle of view does not increase the ability to see polyps and adenomas.

Another study[18] reported a large randomized trial but did not show any objective advantage of the high-definition instrument using narrow-band imaging over the same wide-angle high-definition scope using white light imaging. Only hyperplastic polyps were found to be more frequent in the group for whom narrow band imaging was used. Other investigators[19] using tandem colonoscopy and either narrow band imaging or white light (both with wide-angle high-definition instruments) found that the neoplasm detection rates were similar when the mucosa was viewed with narrow-band imaging or white light. The conclusion was that they did not find narrow-band imaging to significantly influence the likelihood of missing or detecting a colorectal neoplasm as compared with white light.

During evaluation of the wide-angle instruments, multiple comparisons have been made to study whether there is any significant difference in cecal intubation with the 170° colonoscope as compared with one with a 140° angle of view. The 2 instruments being compared in several reports were identical in every aspect except for the angle of view. In one study,[13] the mean insertion time to the cecum was shorter with the wide-angle colonoscope than with the standard colonoscope (2.09 vs 2.53 minutes). Similarly, the mean withdrawal time was shorter with the wide-angle instrument (4.98 vs 5.74 minutes) than with the standard colonoscope. Colonoscopists in a dual-center study[15] also looked at the insertion time of a standard colonoscope versus a wide-angle colonoscope. The mean insertion time was similar, and the mean withdrawal time of the wide-angle instrument was somewhat shorter than for the standard colonoscope, 4.9 minutes versus 5.4 minutes, respectively. Another study with the wide-angle instrument[12] determined that its use resulted in a more rapid examination, with the mean time for examination with the wide-angle colonoscope being 6.75 minutes versus 7.64 minutes with the standard colonoscope. During this evaluation the aim was to withdraw the standard or the wide-angle colonoscope as rapidly as possible while yet being able to examine the entire lumen and the proximal side of any fold or structure. The mean extubation time with the wide-angle colonoscope was reduced by 25% to 30% as compared with the 140° instrument. Another report[14] compared the standard colonoscope with the wide-angle colonoscope, and found no statistical difference in either intubation or withdrawal time between the 2 instruments when a minimal 6-minute extubation time was mandated. The reports in the medical literature confirm that the extubation time may be up to 1 minute shorter with a wide-angle colonoscope because of the ability to expose a greater surface area than can be visualized with an instrument having a 140° angle of view. However, this does not translate into a clinically meaningful advantage unless it results in a greater polyp-finding capability. The polyp miss rate has been investigated (vide supra) and there has been no significant difference shown in the probability of missing polyps as adenomas, whether the instrument used had a wide-angle as opposed to a narrower angle of view.

In the continuing quest to find changes in design, techniques, or accessories to make the colonoscopic examination more efficient, a cap or hood in the instrument has been investigated. The use of this device keeps the tip of the scope from contacting the mucosal surface to prevent obstruction of vision when the scope tip is deflected around a fold or a bend in the colon. The cap could be of use to flatten folds and thus see lesions that grow behind folds unseen by standard straightforward colonoscopy. It was the consideration that a clear plastic cap could be used as an extension of the colonoscope's tip while permitting the portion of mucosa that is deflected to be seen through the transparent hood (**Fig. 3**).

Use of a transparent cap to assist in viewing behind haustral folds was suggested in 1995 by Inoue and colleagues.[20] In this article, the cap was reported to avoid contact of the lens with the mucosal surface, and the colon wall could be seen through the clear plastic hood attached to the colonoscope tip. The investigators described that the area behind folds could be observed by compressing the fold to flatten it using the edge of the cap. In 1998 Matsushita and colleagues[21] described in 24 subjects a decreased miss rate for polyps when using a transparent cap as compared with a colonoscope without the cap. This tandem study randomized patients with known polyps to an examination with or without the cap. No polyps were missed when using the cap as opposed to a 15% miss rate with standard colonoscopy. All of the missed polyps were smaller than 5 mm except one of 8 mm diameter.

Using a colonoscope with a transparent hood, Kondo and colleagues[22] found in a randomized control trial of 721 patients at least one polyp in significantly more

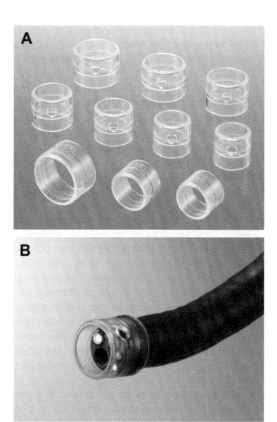

Fig. 3. (*A*) An array of hoods of various diameters and lengths to accommodate different instruments and different procedures. (*B*) A colonoscope with a transparent hood attached to the tip. The side hole in the plastic tip is meant to allow fluid that can collect in the hood to drain out. Hoods may be of different lengths and diameters to accommodate different instruments.

subjects than in those with no hood, but prevalence rates (polyps/patient) were identical. The conclusion of the investigators was that a cap that extended 4 mm from the faceplate of the colonoscope did not interfere with intubation, but its ability to depress folds and reduce the blind areas hidden behind them led to a higher rate of polyp detection.

Horiuchi and Nakayama[23] performed repeat colonoscopy with an experimental transparent retractable extension hood months after initial colonoscopy showed the presence of adenomas; more adenomas were found on the second examination using the hood. A similar finding was reported from this group in a more recent publication.[24] This unique device has the capability to extend or retract a 7-mm clear plastic cap affixed to the tip of a colonoscope. The hood responds to air pressure delivered to bellows on the cap through a long slender catheter attached externally along the length of the colonoscope. Its usefulness is that fluid and debris that collects and pools in a fixed cap can interfere with vision, but retraction of the cap permits complete clearing.

Hewett and Rex[25] performed a tandem study with 100 subjects, reporting a significantly lower miss rate for cap-fitted colonoscopy versus regular colonoscopy (21% vs

33%, $P = .039$). However, it should be noted that there was still a considerable miss rate even when the cap was applied. Improvement in detection was limited to diminutive adenomas (<5 mm), and there was no significant difference in per-patient miss rates in the comparison of the 2 groups.

Not all reports of the transparent cap on the scope show a benefit in polyp detection. In a report of 592 patients by Harada and colleagues,[26] there was no difference in polyp detection rate between the randomized-cap and no-cap groups. Lee and colleagues,[27] in a randomized prospective trial involving 11 endoscopists in 2 centers, found a significantly lower adenoma detection rate with the cap in place during the evaluation of 1000 patients.

In general, the literature on cap-assisted colonoscopy for diagnostic purposes is inconsistent, and this device does not seem to be of universal benefit for locating polyps hidden behind folds or in the deep valleys between haustral folds.

In addition to wide-angle optics, and a cap on the endoscope tip, other innovations and variations have been introduced in an attempt to enhance the ability of the colonoscopic examination to find more polyps (or miss less polyps) during the examination, including an adequate bowel preparation, slow withdrawal time, high-resolution imaging, dye spray, and narrow band imaging. Despite meticulous techniques and new imaging tools, lesions behind the colonic folds may be impossible to see by any addition to the straight end-on colonoscopic examination.

Retroversion of the colonoscope in the rectum has long been considered an integral part of colonoscopy. A similar capability is possible in the proximal colon, but not investigated until recently. The bending capability of flexible instruments has resulted in frequent episodes of inadvertent retroflexion of colonoscopes during attempts to perform intubation to the cecum. It is possible to purposefully perform retroflexion of the instrument throughout various parts of the colon, in a similar fashion to the procedure that is more routinely performed in the rectum during a colonoscopic examination. A comparison was made between 2 prototype scopes and a standard colonoscope to evaluate the effectiveness and utility of performing retroflexion in the colon. The standard commercially available Olympus pediatric colonoscope has a bending section length of 10 cm (Olympus Medical Instruments, Tokyo, Japan). A prototype instrument with a shorter bending length of 6.7 cm was specifically designed for its capability of easy retroflexion and was compared with a pediatric instrument that has a standard length-bending section, but has a tighter radius of tip deflection curvature than a standard colonoscope. With these instruments, cecal retroflexion was attempted, defined as the ability to see the ileocecal valve orifice en face and also to be able to visualize part of the ascending colon in the retroflexed position. The result was no difference in intubation time to the cecum between the standard pediatric colonoscope and the instrument that had the same length-bending section but a tighter radius of tip deflection. However, during the use of the instrument with a shorter bending section, cecal intubation times were longer and more maneuvers were necessary (abdominal pressure/variable stiffness device activation/position change) to intubate the cecum with the shorter tip deflection instrument. The 2 prototype instruments showed a significantly higher rate of being able to perform retroflexion than the standard pediatric colonoscope; there was no difference between them in the success rate of cecal retroflexion. The success of retroflexion in the cecum was 57% for the standard pediatric colonoscope, and 91% and 94% for the prototype instruments. There was a 98% success rate for all instruments for intubation of the terminal ileum. It was thought that the instrument with the shorter bending section, although easily retroflexed in the cecum, took longer to pass to the cecum and was more likely to require additional maneuvers to reach the cecal tip. The consideration was that the very tight turning radius of the bending section along with the shortened tip resulted in difficulty with advancement because the colonoscope was not able to bend sufficiently when pushed against the wall of the colon. From personal observations the author, too, noted that a short bending section made the colonoscopic examination much more difficult, presumably because the short bending section did not permit the instrument to be pulled back and straightened in a normal fashion, since the bending section was too short to bridge across the lumen of the colon and allow the instrument to be pulled back and straightened. Whenever a straightening maneuver was attempted, the short tip failed to anchor itself in the colon, so that pulling back with the tip deflected merely resulted in pulling the instrument out of the colon without straightening.

Another study[28] was performed with similar instruments, but using adult colonoscopes. One of the prototype adult instruments had a bending section length of 13 cm and the other a length of 11.5 cm. These 2 specialty instruments were randomized, with the standard adult colonoscope not being one of the study instruments. In general, there was no difference in the mean time to the cecum or any of the ancillary measures required for passing the instrument. Regarding these adult colonoscopes, the instrument with a shorter bending section could be retroflexed in the cecum more often than the other, but there were no other significant differences noted with either instrument.

Two articles have discussed the removal of colon polyps during retroflexion with a colonoscope. In the first study,[29] the same 2 prototypes of the pediatric type of colonoscope were used. One has a shorter bending section and the other has a tighter tip deflection radius in the right/left direction as compared with the standard pediatric colonoscope. The technique used for instrument deflection was to advance the instrument tip several haustral folds proximal to the polyp (except when cecal polyps were present). The dial controls were used to deflect the tip maximally in both the left and up directions, and the instrument was then torqued in a counterclockwise (left) direction occasionally with advancement of the shaft. Once a retroversion maneuver had been completed, the colonoscope was then withdrawn until the polyp was visualized. Standard polypectomy procedures were used to remove 59 consecutive large sessile polyps proximal to the rectum. Fourteen polyps were removed partially or completely in the retroflexion mode. There were no perforations and no complications related to retroflexion. The polyps removed in retroflexion could only barely be visualized in the forward view and all could not have been removed except by using the retroflexion technique. A similar report[30] detailed 15 polypectomies with endoscopic retroflexion. All of the polyps were sessile and large (average size 38 mm, range 20–60 mm); of these polyps 3 were in the cecum, 3 in the ascending colon, 3 at the hepatic flexure, 3 in the transverse colon, 2 at the splenic flexure, 2 in the descending colon, and 2 in the sigmoid colon. The procedures were performed using a standard Pentax colonoscope (EC3831L; Pentax Precision Instrument Corporation, Orangeburg, NY, USA). The technique for retroflexion was: advance the scope beyond the index polyp, reduce all the loops in the instrument; bend the tip of the colonoscope fully upward; and advance the instrument until the polyp is seen. Scope rotation was sometimes necessary. Standard polypectomy techniques with endoscopic mucosal resection were performed in both forward and retrograde approaches. There were no endoscopic complications.

The investigators of both these reports state that retroflexion attempts should be stopped if the endoscopist feels resistance when bending the tip or when trying to advance the scope. Often, the use of an upper endoscope may be a good alternative especially when retroflexing in the left colon.[30]

A disappointing view of the value of retroflexion in the right colon during screening colonoscopy was published by the Indiana Group.[31] One hundred patients had all polyps removed between the cecum and splenic flexure and then a repeat examination was performed from the splenic flexure to the cecum and back, looking for polyps that had been missed during the original scan and polypectomy. Following the first examination, the cecum was then reintubated and the patients were randomized to a second examination either using a straightforward viewing technique or by using a retroflexed mode. Standard instruments were used along with prototype pediatric colonoscopes with a short bending section or a tight radius of bending curvature of the tip. Retroflexion was readily made in the ascending colon and transverse colon, but the standard adult colonoscope could only be retroflexed in the cecum approximately 40% of the time and a standard pediatric colonoscope could be retroflexed in the cecum approximately one-third of the time when attempted, whereas the prototype instruments could be retroflexed in the cecum more than 90% of the time. The calculated miss rate for polyps/adenomas found in the forward view during reintubation after the initial colonoscopist removed all polyps was 37%/33%, and when the retroflex examination was performed the incidence of missed polyps/adenomas was 38%/23%. In this report, the calculated miss rate on the second examination when performed in retroflexion was numerically lower than when the second examination was performed in the forward view. The explanation proffered in this report was that the retroflexion does not expose the entire colon to view because the instrument may be difficult to maneuver during retroflexion, or that polyps located in hidden positions on the proximal sides of folds are not the principal mechanism accounting for failure of detection during colonoscopy. Although no complications were seen during this randomized study, the investigators cautioned against routine retroflexion in the right colon because of the possibility of complications.

Rectal retroflexion, on the other hand, has long been taught as the "routine" concomitant to a total colonoscopy.[32] There have been few studies on the yield of finding significant pathology during rectal retroversion. An article from the Indianapolis group[33] performed rectal retroversion on 1502 consecutive patients enrolled in a study of several aspects concerning rectal retroversion. Retroflexion was successful in about 94% of patients, but was not performed in 6% because the rectum appeared narrow. During this study, 7 polyps were visualized only by retroflexion (following a careful planned extubation of the colonoscope with special attention to the rectal mucosa right down to the anal verge). Of these polyps, 6 were hyperplastic sessile polyps and 1 was a 4-mm sessile tubular adenoma. Despite this finding, several gastroenterologists are committed to the concept of performing a rectal retroversion before or after total colonoscopy to visualize the area surrounding the dentate line and the distal rectum. Although there have been reports of perforation related to rectal retroversion, and a few reports of closing those perforations with clips, it is the consideration of this author that rectal retroversion should be performed and need not be uncomfortable for the patient. The technique is to withdraw the colonoscope to the anal verge following a total colonoscopic examination. The instrument is then advanced up to the first or second valve of Houston with the apex of the valve placed at the 12-o'clock position in the visual field. The colonoscope tip is then deflected maximally up and the colonoscope gently advanced, usually resulting in a retroflexion maneuver. If this does not work another valve should be approached, which may be on the right or on the left. The tip of the endoscope is then placed on a distal aspect of the valve and with the tip maximally deflected the scope is then advanced gently. Once the U-turn has been made, the right/left control should be locked and moved maximally to the right, and the shaft of the instrument held near the perineum is rotated in a clockwise fashion, while withdrawing the instrument to move the lens closer to the anal verge. Should the patient complain of pain when the instrument is advanced into the rectum, that particular attempt should be abandoned and another fold approached. Patients should not be discomforted by the retroversion maneuver, and if they are, the tip should be moved to a different location for another attempt. Occasionally the rectal vault may be small, such as occurs after radiation therapy to the pelvis, in inflammatory bowel disease, or in slender women who may have an acute angulation just inside the anal verge. During these circumstances, rectal retroversion should not be performed, and if painful, any attempt should be stopped to avoid a perforation.

The main reason that retroflexion is performed by endoscopists is to visualize more of the mucosal surface, especially those areas that are not well seen by direct end-on examination with the standard colonoscope, whether the location of the instrument tip is in the cecum or the rectum.

As noted before, instrument manufacturers have been dealing with the problem of making an instrument that easily retroflects throughout the large bowel, but up to now the major instrument manufacturers have not come up with an instrument that can easily perform forward and backward (retroflexed) views of the colon. To this end, Avantis has developed a small-caliber endoscope that can fit through the instrument channel of a standard colonoscope. The third-eye retroscope (TER; Avantis Medical Systems Inc, Sunnyvale, CA) was developed specifically because of the inability of the standard forward-viewing colonoscope to find all of the polyps that are located behind folds and flexures in the colon during screening procedures.

The TER is a miniature self-contained endoscope that is passed through the accessory channel of a standard colonoscope, and when positioned beyond the tip of the colonoscope permits a retrograde view of the colon (**Fig. 4**). Whereas the standard colonoscope provides an image of the colon in a forward direction, the TER looks backward toward and beyond the faceplate of the colonoscope, visualizing the proximal aspect of folds as the colonoscope simultaneously views their distal surfaces. The disposable TER is a marvel of engineering, with its built-in 180° tip angulation, light source, and video chip being contained in a flexible sheath of 2.5 mm external diameter, with the tip housing the camera being 3.5 mm. To prevent triggering the automatic brightness reduction feature built into the colonoscope, the TER has

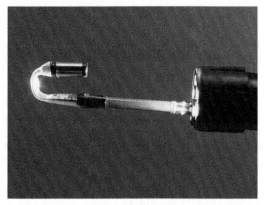

Fig. 4. The third-eye retroscope (TER) flexes 180° to point backward at the colonoscope once it has been extended beyond the colonoscope tip. The video camera and light source bend automatically as the instrument is extended.

a polarized light-emitting diode (LED) matched to a polarized filter affixed to the colonoscope tip before the procedure. This configuration results in the colonoscope light being as bright as usual and not diminished in intensity by the built-in light sensor, resulting in full illumination for both forward and retrograde viewing.

The distal portion of the TER is composed of 3 segments with the camera at the end. When the instrument emerges from the colonoscope tip, the short camera segment bends 90° to sit at a right angle to the long axis of the host instrument. As the device is further inserted into the colonoscope instrumentation channel, the next segment, which contains the LED, maintains its fixed angle with the camera portion and also bends at a 90° angle to the colonoscope. Because the camera segment maintains its right angle to the LED section, it points backward at 180°, bringing it face to face with the lens of the colonoscope and parallel with the colonoscope's long axis, thus resulting in an angulated U-turn. The short section carrying the light assumes its position parallel to the faceplate of the colonoscope. After the obligatory and fixed turns are made as the TER is advanced from the colonoscope's instrumentation channel, the shaft of the TER device is then adjusted to place the camera in a position several centimeters from the tip of the colonoscope. The LED is totally contained in the short second section at 90° to the other 2 segments of the TER, one of which is the portion with the backward-viewing camera and the other being the long shaft of the TER device. The illumination from the LED segment is directed toward the faceplate of the colonoscope and brightens the dark area behind the colonoscope tip. The TER, containing an integrated light source and microchip for visualization, depends on a separate image processor. The images are transmitted by a tiny complementary metal oxide semiconductor chip[34] to the processor and then to the monitor, where side-by-side live video is projected with the colonoscopic image on the left and the TER image on the right.

When the TER is advanced several centimeters beyond the tip of the colonoscope, visualization behind folds and the valleys between folds can be readily observed, providing a complete evaluation of the areas hidden from the forward-viewing colonoscope. Because of the self-contained LED illumination and the 135° angle of view, the previous dark area behind the colonoscope tip can be visualized for several centimeters (**Fig. 5**). The transmitted images from the microchip on the TER and the colonoscope are viewed simultaneously by the trained endoscopist. A CTC simulation model[8] has shown that a retrograde device with 135° angle of view coupled with a standard forward-viewing colonoscope (140° angle of view) will permit almost full optical visualization of the entire distal and proximal colon surfaces.

There have been 5 published reports on the TER. The first was a feasibility study using colon models.[35] Anatomic colon models were prepared for visualization by 6 gastrointestinal endoscopists who used, in a random fashion, a straightforward colonoscope or the same instrument using the TER during withdrawal. These models were implanted with 40 simulated polyps, with 27 of them attached to the proximal aspect of folds and 13 in "obvious" locations readily seen by the straightforward-viewing colonoscope. All the simulated polyps were identical in size, being 3 mm in diameter and 1.5 mm in height, and all were round and brightly colored. Of the polyps located on the proximal aspect of folds, 12% were detected with the straight-viewing colonoscope and 81% were seen with the auxiliary retrograde viewing device. In a subsequent pilot study in humans,[36] the TER was reported to find an additional 11.8% increase in polyp detection as compared with the findings with the straight end-on colonoscope. During this study, a total of 38 polyps were identified in 29 patients as the colonoscope and TER were withdrawn together from the cecum. Thirty of the polyps were seen with the colonoscope, 4 were visualized by both endoscopes (the

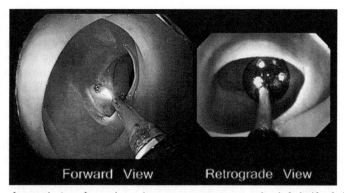

Fig. 5. The forward view from the colonoscope appears on the left half of the display monitor. The retrograde view from the TER is on the right. The TER always looks backward at the faceplate of the colonoscope to illuminate and visualize the areas behind folds and flexures.

colonoscope and the TER), and an additional 4 were seen only with the TER, being located on the proximal aspect of folds. The sizes of these polyps found only by the TER measured 0.3 cm, 0.3 cm, 0.2 cm, and 0.7 cm. All were subsequently seen by the colonoscope and removed. Three were hyperplastic and the largest was a tubular adenoma. The mean time was 22 minutes, which presumably included the time for removal of polyps and replacement of the TER device.

A more recent prospective multicenter study in 249 patients at 8 locations[37] demonstrated an additional 13.2% increase in polyp detection with an 11.0% increase in adenoma detection (**Fig. 6**). During this investigation, 3 additional adenomas whose size was greater than 10 mm in diameter were seen with the TER but not seen with the forward-viewing colonoscope, a 33% increase in adenoma yield when compared with the 9 adenomas of that size that were seen with the standard forward-viewing colonoscope. In this multicenter study,[37] an attempt was made to differentiate

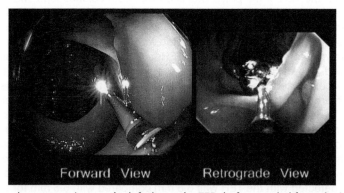

Fig. 6. The colonoscope view on the left shows the TER shaft extended from the instrument channel of the colonoscope. The bright light from the TER is pointed back toward the colonoscope tip. The retrograde view on the right shows the TER shaft extended from the colonoscope instrumentation channel. A polyp is seen by the TER at the 9-o'clock position hidden deep in the crevice behind a fold, not visualized by the forward-viewing colonoscope.

whether polyps seen during this investigation were first identified by the colonoscope or first identified by the TER. Most of the 257 polyps were visualized simultaneously with both the forward-viewing colonoscope and the TER. Those initially seen with the TER but readily apparent on the forward view of the colonoscope were not considered "additional polyps detected by TER." Thirty-four out of 257 polyps were considered seen first by the TER. Of adenomas, 15 out of a total of 136 were first seen by the TER. In this group of adenomas, 8 out of a total of 40 adenomas greater than 6 mm in diameter were first seen by the TER (25% yield) and 3 out of 12 were larger than 10 mm. The mean size of adenomas detected with the TER was 5.2 mm compared with 4.4 mm for those detected with the colonoscope. The mean size of all polyps detected with the TER was 4.6 mm compared with 4.2 mm for those detected with the colonoscope alone. Of the 34 polyps detected with the TER, 10 were greater than 6 mm and 4 were greater than 10 mm in diameter. The withdrawal phase of the colonoscope and TER was 10.9 minutes, eliminating the time required for polyp removal. These findings strikingly demonstrate that polyps may be located in areas difficult to detect by forward-viewing colonoscopy. Colonoscopy is the best imaging device currently available for the large bowel, but may be an imperfect tool against colon cancer. Because recent guidelines[38–41] for colorectal cancer screening and surveillance depend on whether polyps were found on colonoscopy and on their size, the need to identify all the neoplasia in the colon has assumed greater importance.

The other major study recently published concerning the impact of experience with the TER on adenoma detection rates[42] demonstrated, in a multicenter prospective study, that the TER increases polyp detection and that the learning curve for its use is relatively short. Fifteen endoscopists at 9 sites participated in a prospective study to determine whether experience with the TER increases both polyp detection rates and procedure efficiency. The participating endoscopists in this study had no previous experience with the TER. Subjects were enrolled, and the initial aim was to have each endoscopist complete 20 procedures. The TER was inserted through the accessory channel of the colonoscope once the tip of the instrument reached the cecum. All polyps found during colonoscopic insertion were removed. During this study, when a polyp was seen the endoscopist indicated whether it could have been seen with the colonoscope using a routine withdrawal technique, or if it could only have been detected with the TER. If the polyp was seen with both colonoscope and the TER, it was credited as being found by the colonoscope. All polyps seen with the colonoscope or the TER were subsequently found with the colonoscope and removed. In these 298 subjects, 182 polyps were detected with the colonoscope whereas an additional 27 polyps were detected with the TER, a 14% increase. The 20 subjects who were enrolled with each endoscopist were divided into quartiles, that is, the first 5 procedures constituted the first quartile, the second 5 the second quartile, and so forth. The learning curve was evaluated by comparing results among quartiles. For all polyps, the additional detection rate for the TER was 17.8% in the first quartile and 17% in the fourth quartile. For adenomas, the additional detection rate using the TER increased from 15.4% in the first quartile to 25% in the fourth quartile. The mean estimated size of all polyps detected with the TER was 6.5 mm, compared with 5.5 mm for those detected with the colonoscope alone. The mean size of adenomas detected with the TER was 6.8 mm compared with 6.5 mm for adenomas found with the colonoscope. The TER allowed detection of 19% additional adenomas with a size of 10 mm or larger. These results suggest that there is a trend toward improvement of adenoma detection with increasing experience, but that all endoscopists learn the basic mechanical skills in the first quartile of procedures, although they did require varying amounts of experience to develop optimal technique.

The technique that is used for retrograde viewing with the TER involves the following:

- Meticulous cleansing of fluid pools in the colon during intubation is necessary, because the TER decreases the suction capacity of the standard colonoscope when it is positioned within the instrument/accessory channel of the standard colonoscope.
- When the cecum has been intubated with the standard colonoscope, the instrument is withdrawn several centimeters to allow safe insertion of the TER.
- A locking mechanism permits stabilization of the tip of the TER once the tip of the TER has exited the instrument channel, and automatically flexes 180%. The TER does not have any controls for tip deflection, but can be rotated to permit cleansing of the lens with the water jet from the "mother" colonoscope.
- The TER and the colonoscope are withdrawn simultaneously using standard colonoscopic techniques. All polyps initially found with the TER were subsequently located and removed with the standard colonoscope in the 2 large published trials.
- During withdrawal, the examiner has to pay strict attention to the side-by-side images on the monitor showing forward and retrograde views of the colon. The eyes must shift between the 2 images, which is not difficult once acclimated to the double image, which are immediately adjacent to each other.
- When negotiating the sigmoid colon, the TER is positioned closer to the faceplate of the instrument because of the multiple folds that would obscure vision of the TER if it remained in the extended mode several centimeters beyond the tip of the colonoscope.

Multiple techniques have been tried in order to enhance the ability to locate polyps during the colonoscopic examination. Multiple studies have shown that increasing the angle of view of the colonoscope has not been of benefit in increasing detection of polyps. In fact, when the angle of view becomes too wide, the ability to detect polyps may actually decrease. There are mixed results when adding a cap to the colonoscope tip. The TER appears to be a useful device to visualize "hidden" colon polyps that cannot be seen by the straightforward-viewing colonoscope. The overall expected increase in rate of detection of polyps is 11% to 13%. Using a single-channel instrument, it is evident that when polyps are found with the TER, the device must be removed from the colonoscope and a snare introduced, and after the polyp is resected the TER is reinserted. Although this is a tedious process, the positive results for an increased polyp detection rate indicate that the TER is currently the best and most effective way of discovering all, or almost all of the neoplasms present within the large bowel.

REFERENCES

1. Lieberman D. Colonoscopy: as good as gold? Ann Intern Med 2004;141:401–3.
2. Hixson LJ, Fennerty MB, Sampliner RE, et al. Prospective blinded trial of the colonoscopic miss-rate of large colorectal polyps. Gastrointest Endosc 1991;37: 125–7.
3. Rex DK, Cutler CS, Lemmel GT, et al. Colonoscopic miss rates of adenomas determined by back-to-back colonoscopies. Gastroenterology 1997;112:24–8.
4. Heresbach D, Barrioz T, Ponchon T. Miss rate for colorectal neoplastic polyps: a prospective multicenter study of back-to-back video colonoscopies. Endoscopy 2008;40:284–90.

5. Bensen S, Mott LA, Dain B, et al. The colonoscopic miss rate and true one-year recurrence of colorectal neoplastic polyps. Polyp Prevention Study Group. Am J Gastroenterol 1999;94:194–9.

6. Soetikno RM, Kaltenbach T, Rouse RV, et al. Prevalence of nonpolypoid (flat and depressed) colorectal neoplasms in asymptomatic and symptomatic adults. JAMA 2008;299:1027–35.

7. Pickhardt PJ, Nugent PA, Mysliwiec PA, et al. Location of adenomas missed by optical colonoscopy. Ann Intern Med 2004;141:352–9.

8. East JE, Saunders BP, Burling D, et al. Surface visualization at CT colonography simulated colonoscopy: effect of varying field of view and retrograde view. Am J Gastroenterol 2007;102:2529–35.

9. Pickhardt PJ, Taylor AJ, Gopal DV. Surface visualization at 3D endoluminal CT colonography: degree of coverage and implications for polyp detection. Gastroenterology 2006;130:1582–7.

10. Arber N, Grinshpon R, Pfeffer J, et al. Proof-of-concept study of the Aer-O-Scope omnidirectional colonoscopic viewing system in ex vivo and in vivo porcine models. Endoscopy 2007;39:412–7.

11. Barthel J. Adenoma detection and retroscopy. Gastrointest Endosc 2010;71:557–9.

12. Rex DK, Chadalawada V, Helper DJ. Wide angle colonoscopy with a prototype instrument: impact on miss rates and efficiency as determined by back-to-back colonoscopies. Am J Gastroenterol 2003;98:2000–5.

13. Deenadayalu VP, Chadalawada V, Rex DK. 170° wide-angle colonoscope: effect on efficiency and miss rates. Am J Gastroenterol 2004;99:2138–42.

14. Pellisé M, Fernández-Esparrach G, Cárdenas A, et al. Impact of wide-angle, high-definition endoscopy in the diagnosis of colorectal neoplasia: a randomized controlled trial. Gastroenterology 2008;135:1062–8.

15. Fatima H, Rex DK, Rothstein R, et al. Cecal insertion and withdrawal times with wide-angle versus standard colonoscopes: a randomized controlled trial. Clin Gastroenterol Hepatol 2008;6:109–14.

16. Kliment M, Urban O, Fotjik P, et al. High-definition, wide-angle colonoscopy for adenoma detection—a prospective study. Scr Med 2008;82:226–32.

17. Burke CA, Choure AG, Sanaka MR, et al. A comparison of high-definition versus conventional colonoscopes for polyp detection. Dig Dis Sci 2010;55:1716–20.

18. Adler A, Pohl H, Papanikolaou IS, et al. A prospective randomised study on narrow-band imaging versus conventional colonoscopy for adenoma detection: does narrow-band imaging induce a learning effect? Gut 2008;57:59–64.

19. Kaltenbach T, Friedland S, Soetikno R. A randomised tandem colonoscopy trial of narrow band imaging versus white light examination to compare neoplasia miss rates. Gut 2008;57:1406–12.

20. Inoue H, Tada M, Takeshita K, et al. Colonoscopy wearing a transparent plastic cap—evaluation of visibility and maneuverability during insertion, clipping, polypectomy and mucosectomy. Gastrointest Endosc 1995;41:378.

21. Matsushita M, Hajiro K, Okazaki K, et al. Efficacy of total colonoscopy with a transparent cap in comparison with colonoscopy without the cap. Endoscopy 1998;30:444–7.

22. Kondo S, Yamaji Y, Watabe H, et al. A randomized controlled trial evaluating the usefulness of a transparent hood attached to the tip of the colonoscope. Am J Gastroenterol 2007;102:75–81.

23. Horiuchi A, Nakayama Y. Improved colorectal adenoma detection with a transparent retractable extension device. Am J Gastroenterol 2008;103:341–5.

24. Horiuchi A, Nakayama Y, Kato N, et al. Hood-assisted colonoscopy is more effective in detection of colorectal adenomas than narrow-band imaging. Clin Gastroenterol Hepatol 2010;8:379–83.
25. Hewett DG, Rex DK. Cap-fitted colonoscopy: a randomized, tandem colonoscopy study of adenoma miss rates. Gastrointest Endosc 2010;72(4):775–81.
26. Harada Y, Hirasawa D, Fujita N, et al. Impact of a transparent hood on the performance of total colonoscopy: a randomized controlled trial. Gastrointest Endosc 2009;69:637–44.
27. Lee YT, Lai LH, Hui AJ, et al. Efficacy of cap-assisted colonoscopy in comparison with regular colonoscopy: a randomized controlled trial. Am J Gastroenterol 2009;104:41–6.
28. Kessler WR, Rex DK. Impact of bending section length on insertion and retroflexion properties of pediatric and adult colonoscopes. Am J Gastroenterol 2005;100:1290–5.
29. Rex DK, Khashab M. Colonoscopic polypectomy in retroflexion. Gastrointest Endosc 2006;63(1):144–8.
30. Pishvaian AC, Al-Kawas FH. Retroflexion in the colon: a useful and safe technique in the evaluation and resection of sessile polyps during colonoscopy. Am J Gastroenterol 2006;101:1479–83.
31. Harrison M, Singh N, Rex DK. Impact of proximal colon retroflexion on adenoma miss rates. Am J Gastroenterol 2004;99:519–22.
32. Waye JD. What constitutes a total colonoscopy? Am J Gastrenterol 1999;94:1429–30.
33. Saad A, Rex DK. Routine rectal retroflexion during colonoscopy has a low yield for neoplasia. World J Gastroenterol 2008;14:6503–5.
34. Rex DK. Third eye retroscope: rationale, efficacy, challenges. Rev Gastroenterol Disord 2009;9:1–6.
35. Triadafilopoulos G, Watts HD, Higgins J, et al. A novel retrograde-viewing auxiliary imaging device (third eye retroscope) improves the detection of simulated polyps in anatomic models of the colon. Gastrointest Endosc 2007;65:139–44.
36. Triadafilopoulos G, Li J. A pilot study to assess the safety and efficacy of the third eye retrograde auxiliary imaging system during colonoscopy. Endoscopy 2008;40:478–82.
37. Waye JD, Heigh RI, Fleischer DE, et al. A retrograde-viewing device improves detection of adenomas in the colon: a prospective efficacy evaluation (with videos). Gastrointest Endosc 2010;71:551–6.
38. U.S. Preventive Services Task Force. Screening for colorectal cancer: U.S. preventive services task force recommendation statement. Ann Intern Med 2008;149:627–37.
39. Rex DK, Johnson DA, Anderson JC, et al, American College of Gastroenterology. American College of Gastroenterology guidelines for colorectal cancer screening 2009. Am J Gastroenterol 2009;104:739–50.
40. Davila RE, Rajan E, Baron TH, et al. Standards of Practice Committee, American Society for Gastrointestinal Endoscopy. ASGE guideline: colorectal cancer screening and surveillance. Gastrointest Endosc 2006;63:546–57.
41. Levin B, Lieberman DA, McFarland B, et al, American Cancer Society Colorectal Cancer Advisory Group, US Multi-Society Task Force, American College of Radiology Colon Cancer Committee. Screening and surveillance for the early detection of colorectal cancer and adenomatous polyps, 2008: a joint guideline from the American Cancer Society, the Us Multi-Society Task Force on Colorectal

Cancer, and the American College of Radiology. Gastroenterology 2008;134: 1570–95.

42. DeMarco DC, Odstrcil E, Lara LF, et al. Impact of experience with a retrograde-viewing device on adenoma detection rates and withdrawal times during colono-scopy: the third eye retroscope study group. Gastrointest Endosc 2010;71: 542–50.

Computed Tomographic Colonography: Ready for Prime Time?

Don C. Rockey, MD

KEYWORDS

• Colon • Cancer • Polyp • Computed tomography • Imaging

Computed tomographic (CT) colonography was initially proposed as a method to evaluate the colon for polyps[1,2] and has grown and expanded remarkably over the previous decade. The growth of the new technology and research has been remarkable. There are many specific issues relevant to the test and its performance, which include the following: (1) test accuracy, (2) patient experience, (3) extracolonic lesions, and (4) colon preparation. There are also many new issues related to training. Also, whether the test is ready for widespread implementation is of critical importance.

The major attraction of CT colonography is that it is largely noninvasive (although there are growing concerns about radiation exposure, discussed later) and relatively simple to perform. Perhaps most importantly, because many patients are currently not being offered a colon cancer screening test, CT colonography offers an alternative, and data suggest that some patients who would not otherwise agree to screening may agree to undergo CT colonography.[3]

ACCURACY

The issue of CT colonography accuracy (ie, sensitivity to detect polyps and cancers) has evolved. Early studies examining highly selected populations and small cohorts, typically at high risk for colorectal cancer, revealed relatively high sensitivities and provided the foundation for the development of further studies. Later studies revealed wide variability in accuracy. Many larger single-center studies demonstrated extremely high sensitivities, but several well-publicized multicenter trials reported variable results (**Table 1**).[4–8] Two more recent multicenter[9,10] studies incorporated elements that suggest that if generalizable, the technology and methodology is capable of detecting a high proportion of lesions. Although there are caveats, the field has advanced to the point that it should be expected that the sensitivity for detection of large (>1 cm) polyps is in the neighborhood of 90% and that this is a level that approaches that of colonoscopy. The caveats include questions about

Division of Digestive and Liver Diseases, University of Texas Southwestern Medical Center, 5323 Harry Hines Boulevard, Dallas, TX 75390-8887, USA
E-mail address: don.rockey@utsouthwestern.edu

Gastroenterol Clin N Am 39 (2010) 901–909
doi:10.1016/j.gtc.2010.08.030
0889-8553/10/$ – see front matter © 2010 Elsevier Inc. All rights reserved.

Table 1
Sensitivity of CT colonography in large multicenter trials

	Sensitivity (%)			
	Per Patient		**Per Polyp**	
References	**6–9 mm**	**≥10 mm**	**6–9 mm**	**≥10 mm**
Pickhardt et al,[6] 2003[a]	(n = 168) 89%	(n = 48) 94%	(n = 210) 86%	(n = 51) 92%
Cotton et al,[4] 2004	(n = 76) 30%	(n = 42) 55%	(n = 119) 23%	(n = 55) 52%
Rockey et al,[8] 2005	(n = 116) 51%	(n = 63) 59%	(n = 154) 47%	(n = 76) 53%
Johnson et al,[9] 2008[a]	(n = 210) 78%	(n = 109) 90%	(n = 270) 70%	(n = 76) 84%
Regge et al,[10] 2009[a]	NA	(n = 131)	(n = 173)	(n = 174)

Abbreviation: NA, not available.
  [a] These studies reported sensitivity specifically for adenomas rather than lesions, and in addition, reported sensitivity for adenomas (including cancers) greater than 6 mm rather than from 6 to 9 mm in size.

generalizability. For example, 2 of the studies[4,8] seem to be more generalizable than the others.[6,9,10] Also, for example, readers in some of these studies were highly trained, some studies used specialized preparative approaches, and some studies used specialized software platforms.

The Intermediate- and Small-Sized Polyp

A critical issue continues to surround the sensitivity of CT colonography for smaller lesions. The available literature is relatively clear on this point. The sensitivity of CT colonography is not as good as that of colonoscopy for the detection of lesions smaller than 1 cm (see **Table 1**). There is even greater controversy about the clinical significance of such small-sized polyp. Some investigators have argued that polyps that have sizes in the range of 6 to 9 mm have little potential for intrinsic neoplasia, whereas others have argued that these lesions pose a greater potential for neoplasia.[11–13] The evidence suggests low malignant potential for these lesions, although perhaps the larger question relates to their longer-term malignant potential. Smaller polyps, which have an even lower risk of malignancy, are also controversial. A consensus radiology working group has suggested that lesions that have sizes in the range of 6 to 9 mm could be followed.[14] This group has further recommended a scheme that does not recommend that lesion sizes less than 6 mm be reported at all,[14] whereas other groups recommend reporting of all polyps.[15]

A recent report suggested that should the consensus radiology working group's recommendations for lesions sized 6 to 9 mm be used in a real-world patient population, up to a third of the patients with intermediate-sized lesions would have polypectomy delayed.[16] With so much controversy, it seems that the best approach is to report lesions and to develop natural history data that allow patients and physicians to make more informed decisions about how to manage these lesions.

Bowel Preparation

A critical issue with all current colon-imaging modalities, including CT colonography as well as colonoscopy, is the need for bowel preparation. A fairly robust body of literature has explored the possibility of modified colon preparation.[17–20] Although some reports have suggested that a high sensitivity for large lesions is achievable,[18,21] the bulk of the evidence suggests that the "minimally prepared" technique is likely not ready for widespread use. Nonetheless, this area is extremely attractive because elimination of the need for a purgative preparation could greatly enhance screening participation.

Patient Experience and Acceptability

Several studies have specifically examined patient experience with and patient preference for colon-imaging procedures.[4,22,23] Patient acceptance and tolerance are obviously complicated and are concerned with preconceived expectations, patient education, physician bias, and local practice patterns. Conclusions from published studies are mixed. Some studies have demonstrated that patients prefer CT colonography, whereas others indicate that patients think that colonoscopy is preferable. Regardless, CT colonography is an important area because the way that the test is perceived and tolerated by patients clearly plays an important role in its use for follow-up examinations.

SAFETY

CT colonography is likely to be very safe. Air insufflation has been associated with a small risk of perforation; the reported risk in large series of patients seems to be somewhere in the range of 1 in 2000.[24–26] It seems that perforations occurring in the context of CT colonography are most likely to occur in patients with underlying colon abnormalities, particularly in those with inflammatory bowel disease (ulcerations or other defects in the colon mucosa may tear if stressed). The other situation in which the risk may be elevated is after polypectomy; thus CT colonography should be delayed after polypectomy has been performed.

Perhaps the most controversial area involving putative risk is that of radiation.[27,28] Collective exposure to ionizing radiation in Western populations has clearly risen in recent years, and the footprint is clear. This exposure has been driven largely by medical imaging,[29,30] and it is arguable that CT scanning has become all too common in the population in the United States. A routine CT scan of the abdomen administers a radiation dose of approximately 15 mSv. The dose for CT colonography is less. However, estimating the risk to the individual is difficult and controversial. Some estimates suggest that the risk of developing cancer is substantial, whereas others suggest that the risk is low. It is likely that the risk varies markedly and is greater for women and younger patients.

Reduction in radiation dosage seems to be readily feasible, with studies demonstrating that colorectal lesions can be accurately identified using low-dose protocols.[17,31] Moving forward, it is clear that a major area of investigation will be lowering radiation doses; some current modeling studies have raised the possibility that CT colonography could be performed with essentially negligible radiation doses.[32]

Extracolonic Lesions

CT colonography detects many extracolonic lesions, which have varying degrees of importance (calcifications, gallstones, hernias, bone lesions, abdominal aortic aneurysms, benign and malignant tumors).[33–36] In one recent study, unsuspected extracolonic cancers were identified in 36 of 10,286 patients, including 11 patients with renal cell carcinoma, 8 with lung cancer, 6 with non-Hodgkin lymphoma, and 11 with other miscellaneous cancers.[37] However, most lesions identified by CT colonography are not clinically important. Although it is clear that CT colonography is able to detect many lesions, it is also clear that the widespread investigation of these lesions leads to additional costs. The magnitude of cost is controversial.[38]

NEW TECHNOLOGY

New technology has advanced rapidly in the field of CT colonography. It seems that the technical aspects of CT scanners have now reached a level at which the examination can be performed rapidly and with relatively low radiation doses. New image display techniques are evolving, and multiple different software platforms are currently available. These techniques, for the most part, share more in common than differences. The most disruptive, and likely the most interesting, new technology is computer-aided diagnosis (CAD). CAD is attractive because it may enhance sensitivity and also reduce reader time.[39] However, a consistent theme with CAD is that its use also seems to reduce specificity.[40] This area in general is controversial, and further study is clearly needed.[41,42]

TRAINING

There is now sufficient evidence to indicate that practically any type of learner, including those with little to no experience in the area of CT colonography, can learn how to perform CT colonography.[43–45] Further, these readers can learn to read examinations accurately. However, it is also clear that specific training is required to perform CT colonography.[46,47]

Germane to the discussion about the specifics of training, abundant literature now indicates that, albeit variable, there is a learning curve associated with the process of gaining proficiency in reading the CT colonographic examination. In one study that included teams of a radiologist and gastroenterologist, it was found that accuracy increased after reading 25 cases.[48] In another study, sensitivity improved after reading 50 cases and seemed ideal after interpreting 75 cases.[49] The case threshold of 75 seemed to be important in another study.[50] In a study with nonradiologists (medical students and radiology technologists) after training using a teaching file of 50 cases followed by blind interpretation of 50 cases, the nonradiologists performed similarly to the radiologists and showed improvement in proportion to case volume up to 100 cases.[43]

An extremely controversial issue surrounds the amount of training exactly required to become proficient.[43,51] The American College of Radiology has recommended an extremely aggressive training experience for those who are not already experienced in the performance and interpretation of CT of the abdomen and pelvis.[52] Their recommendations are as follows:

1. Completion of an Accreditation Council for Graduate Medical Education–approved training program in the respective specialty in which they practice, plus 200 credit hours of Category I Continuing Medical Education (CME) in the performance and interpretation of abdominal-pelvic CT.
2. Supervision, interpretation, and reporting of 500 CT cases, at least 100 of which must be abdominal-pelvic CT during the past 36 months in a supervised situation.
3. Education regarding patient preparation, bowel insufflation, and CT image acquisition.
4. Formal hands-on interactive training using dedicated CT colonography software, including the interpretation, reporting, and/or supervised review of at least 75 endoscopically confirmed CT colonography cases using primary 2-dimensional (D) and/or primary 3D search with routine problem-solving techniques.

While the last 2 recommendations seems to be highly reasonable, the first 2 recommendations do not and indeed do not seem to be based on available literature, which suggests that the learning curve for CT colonography is in the range of 50 to 100 cases.

In contrast, the American Gastroenterological Association has proposed the following training specifically for gastroenterologists because CT colonographic interpretation should address cognitive skills required to perform all aspects of the CT colonographic examination (**Box 1**).[53] These recommendations include initial training as well as ongoing training, are rigorous, and readily allow gastroenterologists to read CT colonography examinations. An area of common ground between the 2 groups may exist in that it may be acceptable for a reader with less experience than a board-certified radiologist with expertise in cross-sectional imaging to read the intracolonic component of the CT colonography examination, whereas it may be most appropriate for a more-experienced reader to read the extracolonic portion.

Regardless of who could or should read the examinations, currently, there is a general consensus that there are few adequately trained readers.

IMPLEMENTATION

Perhaps, the most challenging issue of all is whether CT colonography can be broadly implemented as a colon cancer–screening test. For example, although the technique represents an attractive method for colon cancer screening, it is unknown whether placing CT colonography in a list of competing screening strategies would enhance compliance.

In addition, there remains great controversy surrounding the issue of effectiveness of CT colonography compared with other modalities. Some studies indicate that CT colonography may be cost-effective, whereas others suggest that it is not as cost-effective as colonoscopy.[54–57] In most scenarios, CT colonography is cost-effective for colon cancer screening when it is much less expensive than colonoscopy.

Box 1
Training in CT colonography for gastroenterologists

- Gastroenterologists performing and interpreting CT colonography should have a thorough understanding of the indications and the principles and limitations of the technology.

- Formalized training of gastroenterologists for CT colonography interpretation is mandatory.

- Training of gastroenterologists for CT colonography interpretation should address cognitive skills required to perform all aspects of the CT colonographic examination (see **Table 1**).

- Training of gastroenterologists for CT colonographic interpretation should include review and interpretation of at least 75 cases from within a well-described training set with endoscopic correlation.

- Review and interpretation of the 75 cases included as initial training can occur at one sitting or be spread over a period not exceeding 8 weeks.

- After initial training, the gastroenterologist should participate in a mentored CT colonography preceptorship, occurring over 3 months and within 6 months of the review and interpretation of the initial 75 training cases. This preceptorship may be individualized training with a mentor in person or may take place in any of the several scenarios (eg, web-based mentoring) and should involve the interpretation of at least 100 additional cases with endoscopic correlates.

- After initial training and a mentored CT colonographic preceptorship, gastroenterologists should supervise and interpret a minimum of 25 cases per year, in addition to participating in continuing medical education activities, to be updated on advances in the field.

Data from Cash BD, Rockey DC, Brill JV. Standards for gastroenterologists for performing and interpreting diagnostic computed tomography colonography: 2010 update. Gastroenterology, in press.

A critical area with regard to implementation, particularly for gastroenterologists, is how the implementation of CT colonography may affect clinical practice.[58] In one modeling study, widespread use of CT colonography led to a dramatic reduction in the number of screening colonoscopies performed as well as to a significant reduction in the total number of colonoscopies performed.[58] In a real-life practice, it has been reported that CT colonography only modestly affected the numbers of colonoscopies performed.[59] It is clear that if CT colonography simply replaces screening colonoscopy, then the impact on colonoscopy volume will be enormous. At present, one of the most important roles for CT colonography is for it to be attractive so that patients unwilling to undergo colonoscopy might be willing to undergo CT colonography, leading to additional screening. If CT colonography leads to incremental increases in the number of patients screened, then it would complement current standard colonoscopy practice and likely benefit patients.

An issue for gastroenterologists interested in CT colonography is concerned with the actual implementation of the test into their practice. Models have been developed in which gastroenterologists and radiologists work together toward implementation of rigorous screening programs. These models have largely been successful, although they have been hindered substantially by the decision of the Center for Medicare/Medicaid Services to not reimburse CT colonography for colon cancer screening.[60] Despite this decision, some gastroenterologists have taken a lead in the implementation of this technology into their practice and/or their community. However, issues having to do with reimbursement, quality improvement, legal and reimbursement issues, and business models for incorporating CT colonography into the gastrointestinal practice thus remain.[53]

At present, if CT colonography is to become acceptable as a primary colorectal cancer–screening modality, there is concern as to how it could be performed in large numbers. CT scanners are prevalent in the United States, but unfortunately, there are not enough skilled readers to handle the large number of screening examinations that are necessary.

SUMMARY

The current data indicate that CT colonography is a reliable and safe colon-imaging test. However, the answer to the question as to whether CT colonography is ready for prime time is currently unclear. On one hand, from an accuracy standpoint, the test is accurate and compares favorably with other current colon-imaging tests. It certainly deserves to be in the discussion of colon cancer–screening options. However, in 2010, from a practical standpoint, at least in the United States, it is not ready for widespread implementation. The reason is that many questions still remain about its use, for example, the lesion size that should be reported, the handling of extracolonic lesions, who is best qualified to read the test and who should be reading the test, and ways to incorporate CT colonography into current clinical management strategies. The answers to these questions and others are unclear as of now. From a practical standpoint, there simply are not enough individuals who are expert in readying CT colonoscopy to make it a viable screening option. It is clear that CT colonography has great promise, but work remains to be done before it can assume a center position as a screening modality.

REFERENCES

1. Coin CG, Wollett FC, Coin JT, et al. Computerized radiology of the colon: a potential screening technique. Comput Radiol 1983;7:215.

2. Vining DJ. Virtual endoscopy flies viewer through the body. Diagn Imaging (San Franc) 1996;18:127.
3. Ho W, Broughton DE, Donelan K, et al. Analysis of barriers to and patients' preferences for CT colonography for colorectal cancer screening in a nonadherent urban population. AJR Am J Roentgenol 2010;195:393.
4. Cotton PB, Durkalski VL, Pineau BC, et al. Computed tomographic colonography (virtual colonoscopy): a multicenter comparison with standard colonoscopy for detection of colorectal neoplasia. JAMA 2004;291:1713.
5. Johnson CD, Harmsen WS, Wilson LA, et al. Prospective blinded evaluation of computed tomographic colonography for screen detection of colorectal polyps. Gastroenterology 2003;125:311.
6. Pickhardt PJ, Choi JR, Hwang I, et al. Computed tomographic virtual colonoscopy to screen for colorectal neoplasia in asymptomatic adults. N Engl J Med 2003;349:2191.
7. Pineau BC, Paskett ED, Chen GJ, et al. Virtual colonoscopy using oral contrast compared with colonoscopy for the detection of patients with colorectal polyps. Gastroenterology 2003;125:304.
8. Rockey DC, Paulson E, Niedzwiecki D, et al. Analysis of air contrast barium enema, computed tomographic colonography, and colonoscopy: prospective comparison. Lancet 2005;365:305.
9. Johnson CD, Chen MH, Toledano AY, et al. Accuracy of CT colonography for detection of large adenomas and cancers. N Engl J Med 2008;359:1207.
10. Regge D, Laudi C, Galatola G, et al. Diagnostic accuracy of computed tomographic colonography for the detection of advanced neoplasia in individuals at increased risk of colorectal cancer. JAMA 2009;301:2453.
11. Ransohoff DF. CON: immediate colonoscopy is not necessary in patients who have polyps smaller than 1 cm on computed tomographic colonography. Am J Gastroenterol 2005;100:1905.
12. Rex DK. PRO: patients with polyps smaller than 1 cm on computed tomographic colonography should be offered colonoscopy and polypectomy. Am J Gastroenterol 2005;100:1903.
13. Rockey DC. Colon cancer screening, polyp size, and CT colonography: making sense of it all? Gastroenterology 2006;131:2006.
14. Zalis ME, Barish MA, Choi JR, et al. CT colonography reporting and data system: a consensus proposal. Radiology 2005;236:3.
15. Rex DK, Lieberman D. ACG colorectal cancer prevention action plan: update on CT-colonography. Am J Gastroenterol 2006;101:1410.
16. Rex DK, Overhiser AJ, Chen SC, et al. Estimation of impact of American College of Radiology recommendations on CT colonography reporting for resection of high-risk adenoma findings. Am J Gastroenterol 2009;104:149.
17. Florie J, van Gelder RE, Schutter MP, et al. Feasibility study of computed tomography colonography using limited bowel preparation at normal and low-dose levels study. Eur Radiol 2007;17:3112.
18. Iannaccone R, Laghi A, Catalano C, et al. Computed tomographic colonography without cathartic preparation for the detection of colorectal polyps. Gastroenterology 2004;127:1300.
19. Neri E, Turini F, Cerri F, et al. CT colonography: same-day tagging regimen with iodixanol and reduced cathartic preparation. Abdom Imaging 2009;34:642.
20. Zalis ME, Perumpillichira JJ, Magee C, et al. Tagging-based, electronically cleansed CT colonography: evaluation of patient comfort and image readability. Radiology 2006;239:149.

21. Keeling AN, Slattery MM, Leong S, et al. Limited-preparation CT colonography in frail elderly patients: a feasibility study. AJR Am J Roentgenol 2010;194:1279.
22. Bosworth HB, Rockey DC, Paulson EK, et al. Prospective comparison of patient experience with colon imaging tests. Am J Med 2006;119:791.
23. van Gelder RE, Birnie E, Florie J, et al. CT colonography and colonoscopy: assessment of patient preference in a 5-week follow-up study. Radiology 2004;233:328.
24. Burling D, Halligan S, Slater A, et al. Potentially serious adverse events at CT colonography in symptomatic patients: national survey of the United Kingdom. Radiology 2006;239:464.
25. Khan JS, Moran BJ. Iatrogenic perforation at colonic imaging. Colorectal Dis 2009 [online].
26. Sosna J, Blachar A, Amitai M, et al. Colonic perforation at CT colonography: assessment of risk in a multicenter large cohort. Radiology 2006;239:457.
27. Brenner DJ, Georgsson MA. Mass screening with CT colonography: should the radiation exposure be of concern? Gastroenterology 2005;129:328.
28. Brenner DJ, Hall EJ. Computed tomography—an increasing source of radiation exposure. N Engl J Med 2007;357:2277.
29. Smith-Bindman R. Is computed tomography safe? N Engl J Med 2010;363:1.
30. Smith-Bindman R, Lipson J, Marcus R, et al. Radiation dose associated with common computed tomography examinations and the associated lifetime attributable risk of cancer. Arch Intern Med 2009;169:2078.
31. van Gelder RE, Venema HW, Florie J, et al. CT colonography: feasibility of substantial dose reduction–comparison of medium to very low doses in identical patients. Radiology 2004;232:611.
32. Flicek KT, Hara AK, Silva AC, et al. Reducing the radiation dose for CT colonography using adaptive statistical iterative reconstruction: a pilot study. AJR Am J Roentgenol 2010;195:126.
33. Gluecker TM, Johnson CD, Wilson LA, et al. Extracolonic findings at CT colonography: evaluation of prevalence and cost in a screening population. Gastroenterology 2003;124:911.
34. Hara AK, Johnson CD, MacCarty RL, et al. Incidental extracolonic findings at CT colonography. Radiology 2000;215:353.
35. Pickhardt PJ, Taylor AJ. Extracolonic findings identified in asymptomatic adults at screening CT colonography. AJR Am J Roentgenol 2006;186:718.
36. Tolan DJ, Armstrong EM, Chapman AH. Replacing barium enema with CT colonography in patients older than 70 years: the importance of detecting extracolonic abnormalities. AJR Am J Roentgenol 2007;189:1104.
37. Pickhardt PJ, Kim DH, Meiners RJ, et al. Colorectal and extracolonic cancers detected at screening CT colonography in 10,286 asymptomatic adults. Radiology 2010;255:83.
38. Flicker MS, Tsoukas AT, Hazra A, et al. Economic impact of extracolonic findings at computed tomographic colonography. J Comput Assist Tomogr 2008;32:497.
39. Halligan S, Altman DG, Mallett S, et al. Computed tomographic colonography: assessment of radiologist performance with and without computer-aided detection. Gastroenterology 2006;131:1690.
40. Dachman AH, Obuchowski NA, Hoffmeister JW, et al. Effect of computer-aided detection for CT colonography in a multireader, multicase trial. Radiology 2010; 256(3):827–35.
41. Petrick N, Haider M, Summers RM, et al. CT colonography with computer-aided detection as a second reader: observer performance study. Radiology 2008;246:148.

42. Taylor SA, Charman SC, Lefere P, et al. CT colonography: investigation of the optimum reader paradigm by using computer-aided detection software. Radiology 2008;246:463.
43. Bodily KD, Fletcher JG, Engelby T, et al. Nonradiologists as second readers for intraluminal findings at CT colonography. Acad Radiol 2005;12:67.
44. Dachman AH, Kelly KB, Zintsmaster MP, et al. Formative evaluation of standardized training for CT colonographic image interpretation by novice readers. Radiology 2008;249:167.
45. Young PE, Ray QP, Hwang I, et al. Gastroenterologists' interpretation of CTC: a pilot study demonstrating feasibility and similar accuracy compared with radiologists' interpretation. Am J Gastroenterol 2009;104:2926.
46. Burling D, Halligan S, Altman DG, et al. CT colonography interpretation times: effect of reader experience, fatigue, and scan findings in a multi-centre setting. Eur Radiol 2006;16:1745.
47. Taylor SA, Halligan S, Burling D, et al. CT colonography: effect of experience and training on reader performance. Eur Radiol 2004;14:1025.
48. Gluecker T, Meuwly JY, Pescatore P, et al. Effect of investigator experience in CT colonography. Eur Radiol 2002;12:1405.
49. Spinzi G, Belloni G, Martegani A, et al. Computed tomographic colonography and conventional colonoscopy for colon diseases: a prospective, blinded study. Am J Gastroenterol 2001;96:394.
50. Thomeer M, Carbone I, Bosmans H, et al. Stool tagging applied in thin-slice multi-detector computed tomography colonography. J Comput Assist Tomogr 2003;27:132.
51. Rockey DC, Barish M, Brill JV, et al. Standards for gastroenterologists for performing and interpreting diagnostic computed tomographic colonography. Gastroenterology 2007;133:1005.
52. McFarland EG, Fletcher JG, Pickhardt P, et al. ACR colon cancer committee white paper: status of CT colonography 2009. J Am Coll Radiol 2009;6:756.
53. Cash BD, Rockey DC, Brill JV. Standards for gastroenterologists for performing and interpreting diagnostic computed tomography colonography: 2010 update. Gastroenterology, in press.
54. Hassan C, Zullo A, Laghi A, et al. Colon cancer prevention in Italy: cost-effectiveness analysis with CT colonography and endoscopy. Dig Liver Dis 2007;39:242.
55. Hur C, Chung DC, Schoen RE, et al. The management of small polyps found by virtual colonoscopy: results of a decision analysis. Clin Gastroenterol Hepatol 2007;5:237.
56. Pickhardt PJ, Hassan C, Laghi A, et al. Small and diminutive polyps detected at screening CT colonography: a decision analysis for referral to colonoscopy. AJR Am J Roentgenol 2008;190:136.
57. Vijan S, Hwang I, Inadomi J, et al. The cost-effectiveness of CT colonography in screening for colorectal neoplasia. Am J Gastroenterol 2007;102:380.
58. Hur C, Gazelle GS, Zalis ME, et al. An analysis of the potential impact of computed tomographic colonography (virtual colonoscopy) on colonoscopy demand. Gastroenterology 2004;127:1312.
59. Schwartz DC, Dasher KJ, Said A, et al. Impact of a CT colonography screening program on endoscopic colonoscopy in clinical practice. Am J Gastroenterol 2007;102:1.
60. Cash BD. CMS's landmark decision on CT colonography. N Engl J Med 2009;361:1316; author reply 1317.

Molecular Imaging: Interaction Between Basic and Clinical Science

Raja Atreya, MD, Maximilian J. Waldner, MD,
Markus F. Neurath, MD*

KEYWORDS

- Endoscopy • Fluorescent-labeled biomarkers
- Endomicroscopy • Molecular imaging

In the past decades, enormous progress has been made in unraveling the pathogenesis of malignant and inflammatory disorders of the gastrointestinal tract. The endeavors taken by scientists are reflected by the successful identification of specific cellular proteins critically involved in the immunopathogenesis of these diseases. These proteins have a decisive effect on the pathologic signaling pathways that lead to uncontrolled cellular proliferation, migration, and aberrant invasion or heightened resistance to apoptosis.[1] These insights in basic science have rapidly been transferred from the laboratory to clinical implementation.

The most prominent application to make clinical use of the molecular insights gained by scientific research is reflected by the evolving diagnostic possibilities in immunohistochemistry, which subsumes diverse methods aimed at recognizing antigens in situ by means of labeled antibodies. Immunohistochemistry is based on the detection of a target antigen in cell and tissue preparations through the initial binding reaction of specific antibodies against the corresponding antigen. To make this immune reaction visible, a fluorochrome is conjugated to the antibody, which in turn is activated through a light source using excitation wavelengths maximally absorbed by the fluorochrome, leading to an immunofluorescence emission that can be evaluated under the microscope.[2] The most commonly used labels for fluorescent immunohistochemistry are fluorescein isothiocyanate emitting green fluorescence or rhodamine conjugates that emit orange to red fluorescence. Immunohistochemistry in tissue preparations has consequently been established in clinical practice regarding

R. Atreya covers a Professorship at the University of Erlangen-Nuremberg which is supported by a grant from Abbott GmbH & Co KG. M.J.W. have nothing to disclose.

M.F.N. provides expert scientific advice to Giuliani Pharma, Schering-Plough, Essex, Abbott, Pentax.

Medical Clinic I, University of Erlangen-Nuremberg, Ulmenweg 18, 91056 Erlangen, Germany
* Corresponding author.
E-mail address: markus.neurath@uk-erlangen.de

structural and functional imaging at the cellular level, as well as regarding diagnostic properties, prognostic evaluation, and even pretherapeutic assessments.[3] This development is especially visible in the setting of gastrointestinal oncology in which tagged antibodies directed against tumor-specific antigens are routinely used in clinical practice to stage and grade malignant lesions.[4] The importance of this field is further emphasized by the advent of novel therapeutic strategies based on molecular targeted therapies that are based on a sound pathophysiological rationale.

The necessity for a sustained therapeutic response, which can only be the result of a more comprehensive approach in targeting critical steps of signal transduction pathways, is best reflected by new therapies not only in oncology but also to a lesser extent in inflammatory conditions. Examples for these molecular targeted therapies are antibodies directed against the epidermal growth factor receptor (EGFR) in colorectal carcinoma[5] or anti-tumor necrosis factor antibodies in inflammatory bowel diseases.[6,7] In conjunction with these therapeutic concepts, the need for molecular imaging methods increases as well.

However, ex vivo histopathologic examination of tissue preparations only offers a momentary snapshot, reflecting the instance where the biopsy specimen is taken from the mucosa, thereby negating dynamic processes taking place in the tissue. Furthermore, the antigen is removed from its natural surroundings and its immunologic activity could therefore be significantly altered. The various fixation and staining processes, which the mucosal specimen is subjected to while the histopathologic section is made, represent another source that could severely influence the expression of the examined antigen. Besides these limitations, the possible risk of physical bleeding and other complications while taking a mucosal sample give reason for the need of alternative methods for nondestructive in situ molecular imaging.

Various imaging modalities have subsequently been used in the past years in different preclinical or clinical settings to evaluate molecular processes in vivo and have given the possibility to analyze the feasibility of various approaches.

Positron emission tomography (PET) and single-photon emission computed tomography (SPECT) have shown considerable promise in this regard and have been used for human molecular imaging for many decades now.[8] The use of PET radiotracers allows the imaging of intracellular molecular processes known to be present during malignancy and thereby enables the localization of primary tumors and metastatic foci in the gastrointestinal tract. PET radiotracers can also assess the efficacy of targeted therapies on a molecular level. This response assessment is therefore beyond the mere evaluation of the size of the tumor because it also takes into account potentially relevant molecular effects, such as anti-angiogenesis, that occur in the initial phase of the treatment. This development is reflected by the introduction of novel radiotracers, which analyze the molecular effects of targeted oncological therapy.[9] A well-established method is the use of fludeoxyglucose F 18 that images glucose metabolism to detect gastrointestinal cancers during PET examinations. The other marker under investigation is ^{18}F 3-deoxy-3-fluorothymidine as a marker for cell proliferation, which might be used in the assessment of early response to treatment.[10] There have also been other reports concerning the use of these imaging modalities for the assessment of response to specific therapies. By using technetium Tc 99m annexin V SPECT to visualize the rate of apoptotic intestinal cells in vivo, it was recently demonstrated that treatment with the anti-tumor necrosis factor antibody infliximab induces apoptosis in lamina propria mononuclear cells in patients with active Crohn disease. Moreover, the induction of apoptosis in intestinal cells also correlated with the clinical efficacy of this treatment.[11]

Nevertheless, there is still the need for the introduction of optical molecular imaging in endoscopic procedures, because only this examination provides real-time image information in vivo coupled with the possibility to intervene in the gastrointestinal tract during the identification of the mucosal lesion and can thus be used instantly for molecular targeted procedure guidance. Advances in optical devices, refined biologically derived materials, innovative fluorochromes- and novel conjugation techniques contribute to the recent advances made in this field of molecular imaging and give reasonable hope for improved diagnosis and targeted therapies in gastrointestinal diseases.[12] The following sections provide an overview of the diagnostic and therapeutic potential of optical molecular imaging in the gastrointestinal tract.

MOLECULAR IMAGING IN GASTROINTESTINAL ENDOSCOPY
Instruments for Molecular Imaging

During the last few years there have been tremendous advancements in optical and mechanical technologies for imaging in the gastrointestinal tract. Since the implementation of flexible fiberoptics in endoscopic devices, gastrointestinal imaging has advanced to include video imaging and lately, high-definition systems. Further developments led to image-enhancing methods such as chromoendoscopy, which depicts the topical application of different intravital dyes (methylene blue, indigo carmine) onto the mucosal surface to contrast pathologic lesions against the normal mucosa. The introduction of virtual chromoendoscopy, such as narrow band imaging, or other surface-enhancement modalities improved this development by increasing the contrast between normal and altered tissue.[13]

Although these innovations greatly improved endoscopic possibilities, several studies have shown that in screening and surveillance examinations of the gastrointestinal tract there is still a significant rate of undetected pathologic lesions in the mucosa.[14] Therefore, molecular imaging in the context of endoscopic examinations of the gastrointestinal tract aims at the identification and characterization of mucosal lesions in vivo based on the lesions' molecular composition rather than their morphologic structure alone. Further initiatives to increase the optical contrast in endoscopic examinations are based on using endogenous fluorescence or exogenously applied fluorochromes.

Autofluorescence imaging uses the effect that a tissue that is exposed to light of a defined wavelength responds by emission of light of a longer wavelength because of the excitation of endogenous fluorophores. Dysplastic tissue has an altered composition of endogenous fluorophores and therefore- exhibits a changed autofluorescence spectrum resulting in false-colored images that distinguish themselves from the background of the healthy mucosa. Nevertheless, recent trials showed that this method was not able to significantly improve the diagnostic outcome in the detection of mucosal pathologies, such as adenoma.[15] Contrastingly, another study found a lower neoplasia miss rate in patients with ulcerative colitis compared with standard white light endoscopy.[16] Further studies are required to fully evaluate this technique in screening endoscopies. The limitation of this endoscopic procedure however, is its low specificity and therefore the high false-positive rate in the detection of mucosal lesions. Tissue alterations are not specific for certain pathologies, and inflamed mucosa severely affects the specificity of depicting neoplastic changes.

Further technological advances are reflected by various means of increased magnification of the tissue during endoscopic procedures. This development has culminated in the emergence of confocal laser endomicroscopy (CLE), which is a powerful tool for performing real-time in vivo imaging in the mucosal tissue at the cellular and subcellular levels.[17] This endoscopic technique not only incorporates the benefits of high-resolution imaging of confocal microscopy but also enables subsequent in situ immunofluorescence staining or other fluorescent labeling techniques. At present, 2 CLE-based systems are available, consisting of an integrated endoscopy system and a probe-based system. The integrated system consists of a conventional white light endoscope in which a confocal fluorescence microscope has been integrated into the distal tip. The system uses a 488-nm wavelength laser and enables the detection of fluorescence between 205- and 585-nm wavelengths. The variable imaging depth ranges from the surface to 250 μm.

The flexible probe-based systems are compatible with the working channels of the different endoscopic devices and use blue laser excitation and fluorescence detection over 505 nm. All the commercially available probes have varying imaging planes, which are mostly fixed in each probe and cannot be adapted. The range of these planes lies between 40 and 350 μm.[18] CLE mandates the use of fluorescent agents to enhance contrast, and most of the trials performed so far have successfully used intravenous fluorescein sodium to enhance contrast.

Imaging Agents

The choice of the appropriate imaging agent is based on its molecular size, stability, safety profile, and the specific spectral characteristics of the fluorochrome. Fluorescein and indocyanine green have both been approved for use in humans and exhibit different emission wavelengths.[19] Whereas fluorescein emits green fluorescence, indocyanine green is characterized by near-infrared fluorescence. Indocyanine green has only limited use in molecular imaging because it is difficult to be conjugated with other substances. Therefore, fluorescein is clearly the most widely used fluorescent agent because it can easily be attached to various protein structures. The emission wavelengths of fluorescein are set in the range of 520 to 530 nm during stimulation by lasers at wavelengths of 465 to 490 nm. Adverse events caused by fluorescein usage in humans are rare, and the overall safety profile of this substance in the numerous studies performed so far has been convincing.[20]

Route of Application

There are 2 primary possible routes for the application of the agent for optical molecular imaging.[19] Topical spraying of the substance onto the mucosal surface has been the most widely used method so far because it has many advantages compared to intravenous administration. The relatively large size of the molecular agent used usually prevents it from being able to pass through the epithelial barrier, and thereby, the exposition of the patient to systemic concentrations of the imaging agent is relatively low. Thus, topical application obviously greatly minimizes the risk of possible adverse events and side effects in comparison to intravenous administration. On the other side, there is still the risk for the occurrence of local reactions of the mucosa to the imaging agent, and therefore, the examined area has to be closely monitored for some time after topical application has taken place. Topical application is more feasible because the agent can normally be applied during or right before the imaging procedure, whereas intravenous application requires a preliminary lead time for the agent to get distributed throughout the body has taken place. Topical application of the agent, usually administered via a standard spraying catheter, is not reasonable for use in large mucosal surfaces but is efficient if a region of interest has been identified before, where the agent can be specifically be applied to. Topical administration of the agent requires the target to be expressed on the luminal surface of the tissue or at least to be rapidly accessible by the agent to ensure that the necessary binding reaction takes place.

Intravenous administration seems favorable if subsurface target structures have to be reached and an even distribution throughout the body is intended. Topical application seems to be advantageous concerning safety issues and if the target structure is expressed on the mucosal surface. Nevertheless, there are no molecular substances that have been approved for in vivo use in gastrointestinal endoscopy at present. Because the usage of radiolabeled probes for molecular imaging has become an integral diagnostic part in nuclear medicine, similar developments seem imaginable for endoscopic procedures as well, and current research activities are centered on the development of fluorescent-labeled probes for this setting.

Classes of Targeting Ligands

There are different groups of targeting ligands that are generally possible for molecular imaging modalities. The choice of the appropriate molecular probe depends on the target structure, the specificity of its signal, and its safety profile.[12]

Antibodies are the obvious choice because they bind to their corresponding target structure in a highly selective manner and can be specifically developed against the epitopes of the antigen of interest. Antibodies are well established in the diagnostic field and labeling procedures with fluorescent agents, which are a prerequisite for molecular imaging and a common practice in in vivo preclinical imaging. Moreover, novel treatment regimens with monoclonal antibodies have evolved around the basic concept of targeting specific molecules that have a pivotal pathogenic role in the disease. Consequently, monoclonal antibodies have proved their clinical efficacy for a steadily increasing number of indications and thus have become a major asset in the therapeutic regime of various diseases. Because the biologic relevance of these targets has already been established, monoclonal antibodies already approved for therapeutic use represent an attractive targeting ligand in molecular imaging. It is conceivable that the intensity of the binding reaction of the antibody to the mucosal lesion could potentially predict the response to this therapy. In this case, the individual "antibody against the molecular target" binding saturation would directly correlate with the therapeutic efficacy of the substance.[21] This approach is especially attractive in the prediction of response to targeted chemotherapy for malignant disorders and could therefore have direct therapeutic consequences, because it enables the stratification of patients before the initiation of the intended therapy. The high binding affinity for the defined target is another advantage of antibodies in molecular imaging because it minimizes the unspecific background signal. On the other hand, most of the used antibodies have a certain immunogenic property that may confer allergic reactions, especially after systemic application. The long half-life of these antibodies in blood may have an effect on the specificity of the signal, because systemic application could lead to the accumulation of the labeled antibodies and hence a heightened unspecific background signal. The high molecular weight and size of labeled antibodies lead to a slow and restricted delivery to the intended target structure, limiting its usage in systemic applications. Therefore, labeled antibodies are probably best used via topical application for the visualization of extracellular molecular targets expressed on the cellular surface.

Several novel approaches aim at formulating molecular probe classes that might be able to overcome the limitations of molecular imaging via labeled antibodies. The generation of antibody fragments has led to a significant reduction in the ligand size, resulting in improved clearance times while retaining high binding affinity to the target structure. Targeting peptides are a further development in molecular imaging because they consist of only few amino acids that have high target affinity and specificity, with even shorter blood clearance times. These peptides therefore have low immunogenic properties and seem suitable for topical administration in molecular imaging procedures. The so-called small molecules that are loaded with various proteins for stronger target recognition are other possible alternatives because they exhibit high specificity and could even be able to visualize intracellular targets or different targets with the same molecule. Their small size might enable them to penetrate more easily into diseased mucosa, thus potentially binding to molecular targets at greater tissue depths. However the conjugation of these small molecules with adequate fluorochromes increases its total size and could affect the biodistribution of the labeled molecule. Potential toxicologic effects of nonbiocompatible structures of these small molecules are further hindrances that have to be taken into consideration before clinically testing these promising substances for molecular imaging in endoscopy.[19]

All these molecular probes have in common that their mode of action is based on direct binding to the target. This action is associated with the possibility of high background signals caused by unspecific binding that does not reflect the true level of expression of the biologic target. In contrast, refined classes of optical imaging agents have been newly developed, which change their fluorescent properties only after prior target interaction.[22] These smart probes are initially in an optical non-activated state because the close proximity of the fluorochromes on the molecular probe results in autoquenching where almost no fluorescent signal can be detected. After binding to the target structure, the probes are activated by proteases overexpressed at the target site. The ensuing enzymatic cleavage of the fluorochromes results in activation and thus amplification of the fluorescent signal. This activation greatly enhances the signal to background ratio for fluorescent imaging and allows rapid screening of large surface areas.[21] This approach has shown particular promise in preclinical studies exploiting the protease overexpression seen in experimental intestinal adenomas and adenocarcinomas.[22] Another approach in this context are pH-activable probes, which are internalized after binding to target structures on the cell surface of malignant cells and are subsequently activated according to the prevalent pH.[23] Again, the currently undefined safety profile has to be closely evaluated before clinical studies on these substances can be performed.

Molecular Targets

Based on novel findings derived from research endeavors unraveling the pathogenesis of inflammatory or malignant conditions, several biologic targets have been identified that come into consideration for molecular imaging in gastrointestinal endoscopy. The selected target has to be accessible for the molecular probe applied and specific for the gastrointestinal disorder investigated. In this setting, the possible biologic target structures are specific cell surface receptors, proteins in the extracellular matrix, various metabolites, intercellular or vessel structures and even distinctive subsets of cells. The decision which molecular structure or pathway should be targeted in molecular imaging procedures depends on the clinical setting in which the endoscopic examination takes place. Molecular imaging can be used for improved detection of polyps or adenocarcinomas in surveillance endoscopies to increase the contrast between normal and altered tissue. The sensitivity of the chosen target is essential for differentiating malignantly transformed and normal tissue. In situ characterization of already identified mucosal lesions, to determine if the finding is clinically significant and needs immediate handling or not, highly influences the selection of the molecular target because a higher specificity of the procedure is prerequisite.

Another highly attractive application for molecular imaging in gastrointestinal endoscopy is the possible stratification of patients to respond to molecular specific therapies before the initiation of the treatment. Reliable prediction of response to biologic therapies would enable a better selection of suitable patients for treatment beforehand, thus decreasing morbidity in patients with a low likelihood of response and enhancing cost-effective use of these treatment options. This approach assumes that there is a direct correlation between the expression levels of target molecules and the response to the associated biologic therapy directed against it. In this setting, basic science is indispensable because it is able to unravel the molecular mechanism of action of novel therapies to present possible molecular targets for imaging. Another likely approach is to label already approved biologic therapies with appropriate fluorochromes and subsequently quantify their binding reaction to the tissue, which might correlate with the specific therapeutic response. Appropriate selection of proliferation markers in malignant disorders of the gastrointestinal tract could also serve as molecular targets in endoscopic examinations to assess the efficacy of therapeutic strategies at an earlier stage than traditional anatomic imaging used at present.

Clinical studies using molecular imaging in gastrointestinal endoscopy

In vivo molecular imaging has been the subject of an increasing number of preclinical and clinical trials, with the potential to significantly affect basic and clinical science in the field of gastrointestinal endoscopy. In a pilot trial, a fluorescent-labeled monoclonal antibody directed against the carcinoembryonic antigen was topically applied during colonoscopy in patients with colorectal polyps or tumors. The endoscopic procedure was performed using a conventional endoscope in which the optical range was increased via narrow band filters. It was shown that a specific fluorescence signal was present in most carcinomas. This effort served as a valuable proof-of-principle study and enabled further trials.[24]

Further advances were achieved in subsequent animal studies. In an important study, a substrate probe specific for the enzyme cathepsin B, a protease that is known to be upregulated in gastrointestinal tumors, was created and conjugated with a near-infrared–based signal that is quenched in its intact state. After intravenous administration of this molecular probe in mice, the cathepsin B–activated beacon demonstrated a high specificity in detecting even small adenomas during colonoscopy.[22] In another study, this concept was taken even further toward a possible clinical application, when a commercially available capsule was equipped with a filter device capable of near-infrared imaging. In ex vivo studies, this capsule successfully detected and transmitted cathepsin B–derived near-infrared fluorescence signals in mouse models for intestinal polyposis and inflammation.[25] These works demonstrated the possibilities of molecular imaging by capsule endoscopy, and further studies are awaited.

The introduction of confocal endomicroscopy has led to further developments in molecular imaging. In a melanoma mouse model, in vivo confocal imaging with a hand-held probe enabled the visualization of tumor cells after the injection of fluorescein-labeled antibodies against octreotate.[26]

In a landmark trial, neoplastic lesions were detected during colonoscopy, using a labeled heptapeptide derived from a phage library. Through the use of a probe-based endomicroscopic system, it could be shown that the topically applied fluorescein-conjugated peptide did preferentially bind to neoplastic cells with a sensitivity and specificity greater than 80%.[27] In a further study, a fluorescent-labeled antibody targeting the EGFR was tested against human xenograft tumors in mice. In this experimental setting, confocal endomicroscopy could accurately identify EGFR expression. In human tissue samples ex vivo, confocal endomicroscopy was even able to differentiate between malignantly transformed tissue and non-neoplastic tissue after topical application of the fluorescent-labeled antibody.[28]

Own studies used the concept of molecular imaging to visualize the processes of tumor angiogenesis in a xenograft mouse model (**Fig. 1**). Because the process of neo-vascularization has long been identified as an essential step in promoting tumor growth and dissemination, modulation of angiogenesis is currently considered to be one of the most promising therapeutic strategies in patients with advanced colorectal cancer (CRC).[29] Studies on CRC have focused on integrins as targets for pharmaceutical intervention because these adhesion molecules play a major role in regulating cell adhesion to the extracellular matrix and are also directly involved in carcinogenesis and metastasis.[30] The integrin $\alpha_v\beta_3$ is expressed by newly formed blood vessels in diseased and neoplastic tissue and therefore represents a reliable marker for angiogenesis in CRC. It could be shown that the vascular expression level of $\alpha_v\beta_3$ in colon carcinomas has a high prognostic value for overall survival.[31] Therefore, evaluation of $\alpha_v\beta_3$ levels in CRC could serve as a valuable indicator for the course of the disease and may also have direct implications for the assessment of response to anti-angiogenic therapies. Hence, molecular imaging modalities represent an attractive tool for targeted visualization of this tumor-associated molecule in vivo. Therefore, in initial studies, the authors injected SW620 CRC cells into nude mice. After intestinal tumor formation, fluorescent markers for the integrin $\alpha_v\beta_3$ were administered intravenously into the xenograft mice model. Targeted fluorescence signals for $\alpha_v\beta_3$ were visualized in vivo via a full body fluorescent scanner, demonstrating increased angiogenesis in the cancer tissue (see **Fig. 1A**). The vascular endothelial growth factor (VEGF) is another important molecule promoting tumor growth and vascularization in neoplastic intestinal tissue.[32] Subsequently, a monoclonal antibody against VEGF (bevacizumab) was the first anti-angiogenic drug approved for the treatment of metastatic CRC.[33] One of the corresponding receptors for VEGF is the vascular endothelial growth factor

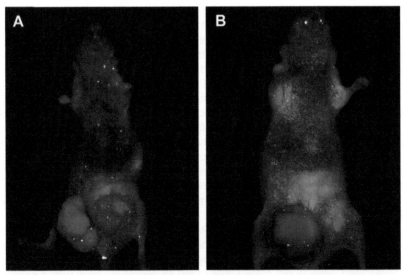

Fig. 1. Molecular in vivo imaging of tumor angiogenesis in mice. SW620 colorectal cancer cells were injected into the inguinal mammary fat pad of nude mice. As the tumors had reached a size greater than 5 mm, fluorescent markers for integrin $\alpha_v\beta_3$ (*A*) or vascular endothelial growth factor receptor 2 (*B*) were injected intravenously, and fluorescence was detected using a multispectral in vivo imaging system (Maestro, Intas, Göttingen, Germany). A strong signal in the tumor region was apparent, representing sustained angiogenesis in the cancer tissue.

receptor 2 (VEGFR-2), which seems to mediate almost all of the known cellular responses to VEGF.[34] Again, in vivo macroscopic imaging was performed in the xenograft tumor mouse model using a fluorescent-labeled antibody against the VEGFR-2 and a multispectral in vivo imaging system (see **Fig. 1**B). Strong signal intensity was observed specifically at the site of the tumor. Foersch and colleagues[35] proved that the targeted visualization of a tumor-associated molecule can similarly be achieved via CLE in fresh tumor specimens of human CRC. After topical application of fluorescent-labeled antibodies against the VEGFR-2, CLE displayed sufficient signal intensity and an adequate contrast in the examined neoplastic tissues (**Fig. 2**). The feasibility of this method indicates that similar data might be obtained in the future while performing CLE in vivo.

The approach of first visualizing suspicious lesions macroscopically using a whole body fluorescence scanner and then characterizing the lesions by targeted CLE based on the lesions' molecular signature exemplifies a possible future diagnostic algorithm in the assessment of diseases via molecular imaging. The combination of specific molecular imaging methods might improve early diagnosis of diseases by visualizing epitopes that are selectively expressed in diseased tissue or follow the response to targeted therapies and identify early responders to treatment.

These intricate studies underline the potential of molecular imaging during gastrointestinal endoscopy and give hope for further developments in this promising field.

OUTLOOK

Important breakthroughs in molecular science during the past years have greatly enhanced the understanding of the molecular mechanisms of diseases and enabled

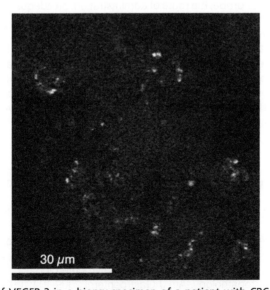

Fig. 2. Imaging of VEGFR-2 in a biopsy specimen of a patient with CRC. VEGFR-2 specific staining with an (Alexa Fluor 488, Carlsbad, USA) labeled antibody against the receptor and visualization via CLE. Intermittent cellular outlines can be observed, depicting different receptor density on the cell membrane. (*Reproduced from* Foersch S, Kiesslich R, Waldner MJ, et al. Molecular imaging of VEGF in gastrointestinal cancer in vivo using confocal laser endomicroscopy. Gut 2010;59:1052; with permission from BMJ Publishing Group Ltd.)

the development of innovative therapeutic strategies. The ongoing interaction between clinical and basic science will provide selective biomarkers that help to establish better overall patient management strategies, stratifying various diseases uniquely for personalized medicine. In parallel, there have been advances in the development of constantly improving endoscopic devices that yield extremely high special resolution and increased depth of penetration, thus enabling the visualization of single cells in the mucosa. These developments form the basis for the advent of molecular imaging in gastrointestinal endoscopy.

The clinical area in which molecular imaging is believed to have a major effect is apparently an increase in the earlier detection of diseases through improved imaging contrasts, differentiating normal and altered tissue. Possible applications include Barrett esophagus, inflammatory bowel diseases and flat sporadic colonic adenomas, which are all prone to the onset of malignant transformation and in which refined endoscopic screening procedures are greatly needed. Furthermore, molecular imaging might enable us to characterize lesions in situ even more specifically, making it possible to stratify different patient groups and predict the response to specific therapeutic strategies. In addition, it is an attractive tool for the study of several gastrointestinal disorders such as inflammatory bowel diseases or malignant disorders in intact microenvironments in vivo, augmenting the knowledge of disease pathogenesis. Even the early assessment of response to selective chemotherapies in gastrointestinal cancers seems achievable because the use of specific molecular parameters (premalignant molecular deviations, angiogenesis, growth factors, tumor cell markers, genetic alterations, markers for apoptosis) could allow the assessment of the efficacy of these therapies at a molecular level before morphologically visible changes take place. The key elements for the successful implementation of molecular imaging in gastrointestinal endoscopy are the identification of the correct molecular target to be imaged and the appropriate molecular probe, the route of administration, an adequate targeting ligand, and a sensitive endoscopic device capable of visualizing the fluorescent signal. Apart from these challenging requirements, the safety profile of the fluorescent-labeled probes is of utmost importance regarding their possible application in humans.

Altogether, the results of encouraging feasibility studies and the anticipated development of new specific fluorescent-labeled biomarkers of disease coupled with novel endoscopic devices pave the way toward clinical translation of the concept of molecular imaging in gastrointestinal endoscopy and give hope for improved diagnosis and targeted therapies.

REFERENCES

1. Terzić J, Grivennikov S, Karin E, et al. Inflammation and colon cancer. Gastroenterology 2010;138:2101–14.
2. Brandtzaeg P. The increasing power of immunohistochemistry and immunocytochemistry. J Immunol Methods 1998;216:49–67.
3. Ramos-Vara JA. Technical aspects of immunohistochemistry. Vet Pathol 2005;42:405–26.
4. Jankowski JA, Odze RD. Biomarkers in gastroenterology: between hope and hype comes histopathology. Am J Gastroenterol 2009;104:1093–6.
5. Jonker DJ, O'Callaghan CJ, Karapetis CS, et al. Cetuximab for the treatment of colorectal cancer. N Engl J Med 2007;357:2040–8.
6. Targan SR, Hanauer SB, van Deventer SJ, et al. A short-term study of chimeric monoclonal antibody cA2 to tumor necrosis factor alpha for Crohn's disease. Crohn's disease cA2 study group. N Engl J Med 1997;337:1029–35.

7. Atreya R, Neurath MF. New therapeutic strategies for treatment of inflammatory bowel disease. Mucosal Immunol 2008;1:175–82.
8. Thakur ML. Genomic biomarkers for molecular imaging: predicting the future. Semin Nucl Med 2009;39:236–46.
9. Josephs D, Spicer J, O'Doherty M. Molecular imaging in clinical trials. Target Oncol 2009;4:151–68.
10. Francis DL, Visvikis D, Costa DC, et al. Potential impact of [18F]3'-deoxy-3'-fluorothymidine versus [18F]fluoro-2-deoxy-D-glucose in positron emission tomography for colorectal cancer. Eur J Nucl Med Mol Imaging 2003;30:988–94.
11. Van den Brande JM, Koehler TC, et al. Prediction of antitumour necrosis factor clinical efficacy by real-time visualisation of apoptosis in patients with Crohn's disease. Gut 2007;56:509–17.
12. Goetz M, Wang TD. Molecular imaging in gastrointestinal endoscopy. Gastroenterology 2010;138:828–33.
13. Wallace MB, Kiesslich R. Advances in endoscopic imaging of colorectal neoplasia. Gastroenterology 2010;138:2140–50.
14. Heresbach D, Barrioz T, Lapalus MG, et al. Miss rate for colorectal neoplastic polyps: a prospective multicenter study of back-to-back video colonoscopies. Endoscopy 2008;40:284–90.
15. van den Broek FJ, van Soest EJ, Naber AH, et al. Combining autofluorescence imaging and narrow-band imaging for the differentiation of adenomas from non-neoplastic colonic polyps among experienced and non-experienced endoscopists. Am J Gastroenterol 2009;104:1498–507.
16. van den Broek FJ, Fockens P, van Eeden S, et al. Endoscopic tri-modal imaging for surveillance in ulcerative colitis: randomised comparison of high-resolution endoscopy and autofluorescence imaging for neoplasia detection; and evaluation of narrowband imaging for classification of lesions. Gut 2008;57:1083–9.
17. Kiesslich R, Burg J, Vieth M, et al. Confocal laser endoscopy for diagnosing intraepithelial neoplasias and colorectal cancer in vivo. Gastroenterology 2004;127:706–13.
18. Neumann H, Kiesslich R, Wallace MB, et al. Confocal laser endomicroscopy: technical advances and clinical applications. Gastroenterology 2010;39(2):388–92.
19. Mahmood U. Optical molecular imaging approaches in colorectal cancer. Gastroenterology 2010;138:419–22.
20. Wallace MB, Meining A, Canto MI, et al. The safety of intravenous fluorescein for confocal laser endomicroscopy in the gastrointestinal tract. Aliment Pharmacol Ther 2010;31:548–52.
21. Mahmood U, Wallace MB. Molecular imaging in gastrointestinal disease. Gastroenterology 2007;132:11–4.
22. Marten K, Bremer C, Khazaie K, et al. Detection of dysplastic intestinal adenomas using enzyme-sensing molecular beacons in mice. Gastroenterology 2002;122:406–14.
23. Urano Y, Asanuma D, Hama Y, et al. Selective molecular imaging of viable cancer cells with pH-activatable fluorescence probes. Nat Med 2009;15:104–9.
24. Keller R, Winde G, Terpe HJ, et al. Fluorescence endoscopy using a fluorescein-labeled monoclonal antibody against carcinoembryonic antigen in patients with colorectal carcinoma and adenoma. Endoscopy 2002;34:801–17.
25. Zhang H, Morgan D, Cecil G, et al. Biochromoendoscopy: molecular imaging with capsule endoscopy for detection of adenomas of the GI tract. Gastrointest Endosc 2008;68:520–7.

26. Becker A, Hessenius C, Licha K, et al. Receptor-targeted optical imaging of tumors with near-infrared fluorescent ligands. Nat Biotechnol 2001;19:327–31.
27. Hsu ER, Anslyn EV, Dharmawardhane S, et al. A far-red fluorescent contrast agent to image epidermal growth factor receptor expression. Photochem Photobiol 2004;79:272–9.
28. Goetz M, Ziebart A, Foersch S, et al. In vivo molecular imaging of colorectal cancer with confocal endomicroscopy by targeting epidermal growth factor receptor. Gastroenterology 2010;138:435–46.
29. Folkman J. Angiogenesis: an organizing principle for drug discovery? Nat Rev Drug Discov 2007;6:273–86.
30. Vonlaufen A, Wiedle G, Borisch B, et al. Integrin alpha(v)beta(3) expression in colon carcinoma correlates with survival. Mod Pathol 2001;14:1126–32.
31. Hood JD, Cheresh DA. Role of integrins in cell invasion and migration. Nat Rev Cancer 2002;2:91–100.
32. Carmeliet P, Jain RK. Angiogenesis in cancer and other diseases. Nature 2000; 407:249–57.
33. Hurwitz H, Fehrenbacher L, Novotny W, et al. Bevacizumab plus irinotecan, fluorouracil, and leucovorin for metastatic colorectal cancer. N Engl J Med 2004;350:2335–42.
34. Holmes K, Roberts OL, Thomas AM, et al. Vascular endothelial growth factor receptor-2: structure, function, intracellular signalling and therapeutic inhibition. Cell Signal 2007;19:2003–12.
35. Foersch S, Kiesslich R, Waldner MJ, et al. Molecular imaging of VEGF in gastrointestinal cancer in vivo using confocal laser endomicroscopy. Gut 2010;59: 1046–55.

Molecular Imaging of Gastroenteropancreatic Neuroendocrine Tumors

Matthias Miederer, MD[a], Matthias M. Weber, MD[b],
Christian Fottner, MD[b],*

KEYWORDS

- Molecular imaging • ^{111}In-octreotide-scintigraphy
- ^{68}Ga-DOTATOC-PET • [18]FDOPA-PET
- ^{123}I-MIBG-scintigraphy • GEP-NET • Neuroendocrine tumors

Neuroendocrine carcinomas (NECs) represent an inhomogeneous entity with growing incidence.[1] They are classified by origin and by functional activity. Also, according to proliferation activity they are graded between highly differentiated (G1) and poorly differentiated (G3) with strong impact on prognosis and therapy.[2] Whereas poorly differentiated NEC is a fast-growing malignancy with generally poor prognosis, highly differentiated neuroendocrine tumors (NETs) may be curable by operation. However, when classified as carcinoma, they always have the potential to metastasize and in an inoperable metastasized stage, cure is generally not achievable with current therapy modalities.[3] Nevertheless, also metastasized, highly differentiated NECs display distinct tumor biology with consequences to the patients. On one hand, highly differentiated NECs are often exceptionally slow-growing solid tumors with courses of the disease of several years. On the other hand, in a significant fraction of patients, the excretion of neuroendocrine peptides leads to disabling symptoms, such as, among others, flushes and diarrhea.[4] These neuroendocrine symptoms may additionally pose a therapeutic challenge in this patient population.

Increasing understanding of the molecular basis of NETs fostered many new targeted therapy approaches targeting, for example, G-protein–coupled receptors such as the somatostatin-receptor (SSTR), intracellular pathways, or angiogenesis.[5] With regard to SSTR expression, highly differentiated NECs generally display characteristic high expression, whereas poorly differentiated NECs might display reduced expression of SSTR.[6] Additionally, variable expression between different origins of

Disclosure Statement: The authors declare no conflicts of interest.
[a] Department of Nuclear Medicine, University of Mainz, Langenbeckstr 1, Mainz 55131, Germany
[b] Department of Endocrinology & Metabolism, I Medical Clinic, University of Mainz, Langenbeckstr 1, Mainz 55131, Germany
* Corresponding author.
E-mail address: fottner@endokrinologie.klinik.uni-mainz.de

Gastroenterol Clin N Am 39 (2010) 923–935
doi:10.1016/j.gtc.2010.08.031
0889-8553/10/$ – see front matter © 2010 Elsevier Inc. All rights reserved.

NEC has been documented by immunohistological and imaging methods with, for example, on average higher SSTR expression for pancreatic NEC over ileum, hindgut, and pulmonary NEC.[7]

Clinically, molecular imaging of neuroendocrine tumors is routinely performed with nuclear medicine methods taking advantage of highly specific radioactive tracers. These tracers are able to depict functional pathways and modern imaging acquisition devices deliver high resolution and ever more quantifiable whole body information. Depending on the decay properties of the respective radioisotopes, imaging is performed by either gamma camera imaging and single photon emission tomography (SPECT) or by positron emission tomography (PET). Both methods are increasingly parts of clinical management algorithms in NETs. Generally, PET imaging is associated with higher spatial resolution, shorter time interval between radiotracer application and image acquisition, and with simple and reliable quantification of tracer uptake (**Fig. 1**). Additionally, hybrid imaging with PET in combination with computed tomography (CT) represents a comprehensive imaging method, increasingly applied in medical centers.

For conventional gamma imaging, the generator nuclide Technetium-99 m (half-life of 6 hours) or the longer-lived isotopes Indium-111 (half-life of 2.8 days) and Iodine-123

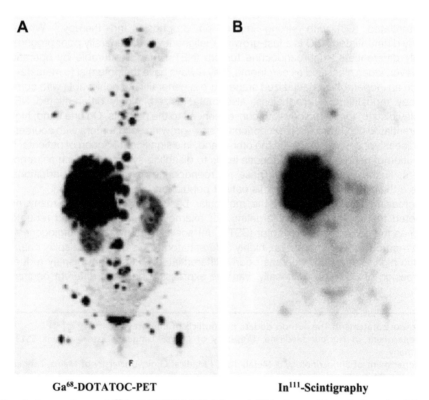

A

B

Ga⁶⁸-DOTATOC-PET   In¹¹¹-Scintigraphy

Fig. 1. Comparison of ⁶⁸Ga-DOTATOC-PET (*A*) and ¹¹¹In-Octreotide scintigraphy (*B*) in a patient with a metastatic low-grade neuroendocrine carcinoma of the pancreas. Maximal intensity projection of the PET shows a larger number of metastases, mainly to the bone, that are not detectable on planar scintigraphy.

(half-life of 13.2 hours) are most commonly used. On the other hand, common positron emitting isotopes are the cyclotron-produced Fluor-18 (half-life of 110 minutes) and Carbon-11 (half-life of 20 minutes) and the generator-produced Gallium-68 (half-life of 68 minutes). With available generator systems, the short-lived isotopes are readily available and the appropriate radiotracers can reliably be produced on site. PET is able to acquire an established quantitative uptake parameter, namely standard uptake value (SUV). SUV is calculated by the absolute radioactivity concentration measured in a distinct volume corrected for patient weight and injected total activity.

Several distinct biological properties of NETs can readily be investigated by clinically available radiotracers. Most importantly, their usually high expression of somatostatin-receptor expression and the development of stable radiolabeled somatostatin analogues has yielded a highly sensitive and specific imaging method by means of receptor imaging. Several somatostatin analogues for PET and SPECT imaging and several suitable radioisotopes are available. Higher sensitivity for PET tracers in contrast to In-111-Octreotid (octreoscan) has been demonstrated.[8,9]

Other tracers are able to display glucose metabolism (^{18}F-fluorodeoxyglucose), amine precursor uptake and decarboxylation (^{11}C-5-hydroxy-typtophan, ^{18}F-Flour-DOPA), and the noradrenaline transporter (^{131}I-meta-iodobenzylguanidine, ^{11}C-hydroxyephedrine).[10–12] Other radiolabeled peptides have also been proposed for imaging and therapy, for example, among others, the gastrin-releasing peptide receptor, the glucagonlike peptide 1 receptor and neuropeptide-Y receptor.[13–16]

Additionally, the route of application, eg, intra-arterially versus intravenously, might increase the uptake of radiotracers offering advantages both for diagnosis and therapy.[17,18]

Selecting imaging methods with highest sensitivity, eg, for screening patients with multiple neuroendocrine neoplasms, with a high likelihood of developing a neuroendocrine tumor, or for sensitive follow-up after initial surgery, is challenging. A variety of emerging morphological methods are available. Highest resolution for detecting liver metastasis is often achieved by MRI or for pancreas tumors by endoscopic ultrasound. Depending on the biologic parameters of the tumors, functional imaging might give more accurate diagnostic results and generally display whole-body information. However, in many cases, functional and morphological imaging deliver complementary information. Thus, hybrid imaging such as PET/CT or PET/MRI will play an important role in the future.

Also, the choice of imaging modalities applicable for therapy monitoring depends on a variety of factors. Because of the slow-growing nature of differentiated NETs and because many therapies are associated with symptom control and disease stabilization, conventional radiologic criteria like RECIST (Response Evaluation Criteria in Solid Tumors) might not be sufficient and other parameters are needed.

SOMATOSTATIN RECEPTOR–BASED MOLECULAR IMAGING

Currently, 5 different SSTR subtypes have been identified, with SSTR-2 being the predominantly expressed one.[19] Different somatostatin analogues with different affinity profiles over these receptors are currently in clinical use or in development. Furthermore, because of different chemical properties of radioisotopes, differences in affinity profiles may also arise between, for example, the diagnostic isotope Gallium-68 (^{68}Ga) and the therapeutic beta-emitting isotope Yttrium-90 (**Table 1**). Somatostatin-receptor targeting is therapeutically used also with nonradioactive somatostatin analogues. To minimize competition for the receptor they should be withdrawn either 24 hours for short-acting somatostatin analogues or 4 to 8 weeks

Table 1
Affinity profiles of somatostatin and currently used radiolabeled somatostatin analogues

Affinity-Profiles of Somatostatin-Analogues (IC50-Values, nmol/L)					
Peptide	SSR1	SSR2	SSR3	SSR4	SSR5
Somatostatin-28	3,8	2,5	5,7	4,2	3,7
Gallium-68-DOTATOC	>10000	2,5	612	>1000	73
Gallium-68-DOTATATE	>10000	0,2	>1000	300	377
Gallium-68-DOTANOC	>10000	1,9	40	260	7,2
Indium-111-DTPA-Octreotide	>10000	22	182	>1000	273

Data from Reubi JC, Schar JC, Waser B, et al. Affinity profiles for human somatostatin receptor subtypes SST1-SST5 of somatostatin radiotracers selected for scintigraphic and radiotherapeutic use. Eur J Nucl Med 2000;27(3):273–82; Antunes P, Ginj M, Zhang H, et al. Are radiogallium-labelled DOTA-conjugated somatostatin analogues superior to those labelled with other radiometals? Eur J Nucl Med Mol Imaging 2007;34:982–93.

for long-acting somatostatin analogues before diagnostic procedures targeting the same receptor when clinically possible.

Somatostatin Receptor Scintigraphy

With Indium-111-DTPA-Octreotide (octreoscan), one of the first commercially available and broadly applied radiotracers in this indication, sensitivity close to 90% could be achieved more than a decade ago.[20] Subsequently, somatostatin-receptor imaging has improved staging and follow-up of patients with neuroendocrine tumors and now has a key role in clinical management algorithms.

The main indications are detection and localization of gastroenteropancreatic tumors, pulmonary carcinoid tumors, adrenal medullary tumors, medullary thyroid carcinoma, paraganglioma, Merkel cell tumor, and meningioma. Sensitivities depend on tumor type and localization. For gastrionomas, VIPomas, and glucagonomas, the sensitivity was found to be between 75% and 100% and for insulinomas between 50% and 60%.[21] Because of increasing advances in molecular imaging, mainly by ^{18}F-fluorodeoxyglucose-PET (FDG-PET) CT, other indications like melanoma, small-cell lung cancer, lymphoma, and others are secondary, unless somatostatin-targeted therapy is an option. Additionally, in preparation for peptide receptor radionuclide therapy somatostatin-receptor scintigraphy also plays an important role in defining radiotracer uptake and extent of the disease.

Physiological uptake by somatostatin-receptor binding occurs in adrenals, pituitary, thyroid, and spleen. Urinary excretion and to a much lesser extent hepatobiliary excretion is leading to visualization of liver, kidneys, bladder, and bowel.

The recommended administered activity is 185 to 222 MBq in adults and 5 MBq/kg in children. The amount of peptide injected is typically 10 to 20 µg.[22] Image acquisition is performed at 4 and 24 hours and for more accurate imaging when significant bowel activity is present up to 48 hours. Besides anterior and posterior planar images of the whole body, SPECT imaging for appropriate regions should be included.

The development of Technetium-99 m–labeled somatostatin analogues improved image resolution and availability. However, in contrast to their Indium-111–labeled counterparts, delayed images of 24 hours and 48 hours are impossible, decreasing sensitivity for abdominal lesions. However, with SPECT and especially in combination with CT the sensitivity of gamma-emitting somatostatin analogues can be improved over planar imaging.[23]

In a comparative study of MRI, CT, and somatostatin-receptor scintigraphy, sensitivity for the detection of liver metastasis was highest for MRI over CT over somatostatin-receptor scintigraphy, attributable to the high spatial resolution of MRI.[24] However, somatostatin-receptor scintigraphy performed markedly better when metastasis reached sizes larger than 15 mm. Also, with high specificity of 88%, high availability, and the possibility of whole-body imaging, conventional somatostatin-receptor scintigraphy still plays the key role in diagnosis of metastasis from neuroendocrine tumors.[25]

Positron Emission Tomography with Radiolabeled Somatostatin Analogues

Several Gallium-68–labeled tracers are applicable with differences in their affinity profile toward different somatostatin-receptor subtypes. However, these differences are clinically secondary and application depends on center-specific preferences.

Labeling of PET isotopes like Fluor-18 ($T_{1/2}$ = 110 minutes) or Gallium-68 ($T_{1/2}$ = 68 minutes) to somatostatin analogues has further advanced somatostatin imaging.[26,27] It has been demonstrated that the higher spatial resolution leads to higher sensitivity on detection of differentiated neuroendocrine tumors (**Fig. 2**).[8,9] Furthermore, the uptake quantification with SUV is a parameter that correlates with somatostatin receptor expression.[28] Although it has not been demonstrated that somatostatin imaging by PET can replace morphological imaging (CT/MRI/ultrasound) when therapeutic efficacy during therapy is assessed, the extent of somatostatin-receptor expression gives complementary information.[29] This holds true especially in the situation when somatostatin-targeted approaches such as octreotide therapy or peptide receptor radio therapy is applied.[30]

Recommended administered activity for Gallium-68-somatostatin analogues depends on imaging time, detector sensitivity, and time after injection. Typically,

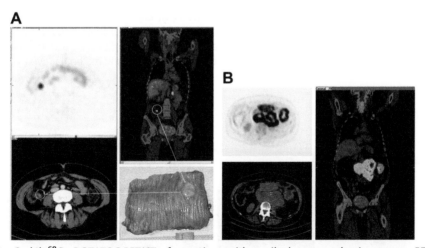

Fig. 2. (A) ^{68}Ga-DOTATOC-PET/CT of a patient with an ileal neuroendocrine tumor. PET demonstrates a small somatostatin-receptor–expressing lesion in the right lower abdomen. Fusion of PET images with CT shows a small tumor in projection to the wall of the terminal ileum. After surgical excision, histologic examination reveals a low-grade neuroendocrine tumor (Ki-67 index <2%) with a maximum diameter of 8 mm. (B) ^{18}F-FDG-PET of a 70-year-old patient with a high-grade intestinal neuroendocrine cancer (Ki-67 index 70%) with a large periaortic tumor bulk and multiple mesenteric lymph node metastases.

activities between 100 and 200 MBq are used with modern PET/CT scanners. Image acquisition is routinely performed 60 minutes after injection, although tracer accumulation is very rapid and some centers use earlier time points starting at 20 minutes postinjection.

Laser Confocal Endomicroscopy with Fluorescein-Labeled Somatostatin Analogues

Recently, laser confocal microscopy has been introduced in clinical routine diagnostics by integrating the miniaturized components of a confocal laser scanner into the tip of a conformité européenne (CE)-certified, Food and Drug Administration (FDA)-approved flexible endoscope. This novel technology allows subsurface histological diagnosis at the cellular and subcellular levels in vivo and provides instantaneous histopathology during ongoing upper and lower endoscopy. Endomicroscopy enables immediate diagnosis of neoplastic and inflammatory lesions of the intestinal mucosa. Previous studies have demonstrated the power of confocal endomicroscopy in screening and surveillance colonoscopy, ulcerative colitis, Barrett esophagus, and gastric cancer and morphodynamic analysis of liver disease in vivo.[31] The integration of a similar miniaturized confocal laser scanner into a handheld device permits straightforward fluorescence confocal microscopy in vivo, allowing exact characterization of cell morphology and dynamic imaging of cellular events identifying various disease states like inflammation, neoplastic transformation, and imaging of microvasculature and perfusion.[32,33] In studies by our own group, SSTRs were used as targets for in vivo real-time molecular imaging using a miniaturized laser confocal microscopy system.[31,34] For selective visualization of SSTR, a novel contrast agent for laser confocal microscopy has been specifically developed by conjugating 5-carboxyfluorescein to octreotate. This fluorescein-labeled somatostatin analogue has been demonstrated to specifically bind to SSTR and exerts a functional antiproliferative effect on SSTR-positive tumor cells. After systemic application, it allows specific dynamic in vivo imaging of SSTR-positive neuroendocrine tumor cells as correlated with ex vivo immunohistochemistry (**Fig. 3**). This not only provides instantaneous high-resolution histopathological tissue evaluation but additionally permits identification and characterization of subcellular molecular structures like somatostatin receptors. In general, the confocal mini-microscopy probe allows the immediate microscopic morphological, functional, and molecular evaluation

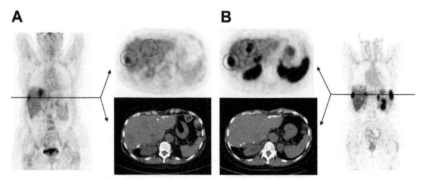

Fig. 3. Comparison of FDG-PET/CT (*A*) and ^{68}Ga-DOTATOC-PET/CT (*B*) in a patient with liver metastases from a low-grade neuroendocrine carcinoma of the terminal ileum. FDG-PET/CT demonstrates partly FDG-positive metastasis with high somatostatin receptor expression, indicating a more aggressive biology, as demonstrated by an increased Ki-67 index of 5% to 10% in a resected liver metastasis.

of all easily accessible organs, thus facilitating screening for and early diagnosis of SSTR-positive neoplasias, because with routine endoscopic diagnostics, intestinal NET can usually not be distinguished from other polypoid structures by macroscopy alone.

OTHER MOLECULAR TARGETS FOR FUNCTIONAL IMAGING OF NETS
123I-Metaiodobenzyl-Guanidine-Scintigraphy

Metaiodobenzyl-guanidine (MIBG) is a norepinephrine analogue that is concentrated in sympatho-adrenergic tissue. MIBG is actively transported through the noradrenalin transporter (NAT) into the cells and deposited in intracellular storage vesicles. MIBG is used as a diagnostic and therapeutic tracer when labeled with Iodine-123 and Iodine-131, respectively. MIBG uptake can be expected in 70% of patients with NEC, where better results are obtained for tumors originating from the pancreas compared with, for example, foregut origin.[35] MIBG shows normally high uptake in liver, myocardium, salivary glands, intestines, spleen, bladder, and thyroid. The adrenal medulla is not routinely visualized. However, faint uptake might be detected.[36] Typically, 370 MBq (^{123}I-MIBG) or 37 to 74 MBq (^{131}I-MIBG, when used for diagnostic purpose) of the radiopharmaceutical is administered by slow intravenous injection. Because of pharmacologic action, several side effects, such as tachycardia, hypertension, vomiting, and abdominal cramps, might occur when the administration of the tracer is too rapid. Several drugs, like antihypertensives and antidepressants might interfere with MIBG uptake either by inhibition of uptake or depletion of storage vesicles and therefore should be withdrawn before the study, whenever possible. Usually, interfering drugs should be discontinued up to 5 biological half-lives before the study. Additionally, thyroid blockade with potassium iodide or potassium perchlorate needs to be administered to decrease radiation exposure to the thyroid. Image acquisition is conducted at least 4 and 24 hours postinjection, preferentially including SPECT imaging.

6-18F-Fluoro-L-DOPA Positron Emission Tomography

NETs are also referred to as APUDomas because of their capacity for amine precursor uptake and decarboxylation. Thus, amine precursors, such as L-dihydroxyphenylalanine (L-DOPA), may be taken up into the tumor cells where they are decarboxylated by the action of the enzyme aromatic amino acid decarboxylase (AADC), which is strongly expressed in neuroendocrine cells and shows high affinity to ^{18}F-DOPA. This reaction converts the precursor into their corresponding amine, dopamine. These are stored in intracellular vesicles where it can be visualized for imaging purposes.[37] Based on the APUD concept, ^{18}F-labeled L-DOPA (^{18}F-L-DOPA), originally used to study patients with movement disorders, has been used in a number of studies to visualize various different types of neuroendocrine tumors, such as medullary thyroid cancer, pheochromocytomas, and paragangliomas, as well as gastro-entero pancreatic (GEP)-NET. Recently, the catecholamine precursor fluorine-18-dihydroxyphenylalanine (^{18}F-FDOPA) has mainly been used as a PET-tracer for imaging of pheochromocytomas and paragangliomas.[38] The advantages of this technique are a quick performance within 2 hours, superior spatial resolution, no interference with medications, and no relevant physiological tracer uptake in normal adrenal medulla. Several smaller studies showed an excellent sensitivity equivalent or superior to the routinely used ^{123}I-MIBG scintigraphy in patients with known or suspected benign and malignant pheochromocytomas and paragangliomas.[39] A recent study of our own group demonstrated that FDOPA-PET is clearly superior to ^{123}I-MIBG scintigraphy in patients with extra-adrenal, predominantly noradrenaline-secreting and hereditary types of pheochromocytomas or paragangliomas. Immunohistochemical analysis of vesicular monoamine transporters (VMAT) type 1 and 2, which are responsible for the specific transport and storage into vesicles, demonstrated a lack of VMAT-1 expression in all MIBG-negative tumors.[12] The lack of VMAT-1 expression predicted negativity for MIBG scintigraphy but not for DOPA-PET, which was positive in all cases (**Fig. 4**). For functional imaging of GEP-NET, DOPA-PET has been used in a number of studies, mainly to evaluate an alternative imaging modality for functioning tumors that are negative on somatostatin-receptor imaging. An initial study by Hoegerle and colleagues[40] reported that DOPA-PET allowed the detection of a higher number of NET lesions in the gastrointestinal tract as compared with SSTR imaging and FDG-PET, respectively. In another study with 22 patients with morphological (CT) and/or biochemical diagnosis of endocrine pancreatic tumors, DOPA-PET allowed the visualization of 50% of the tumors but failed to detect nonfunctioning tumors and small insulinomas. In this study,

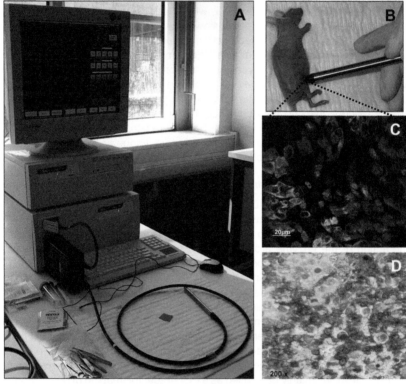

Fig. 4. The miniaturized laser confocal microscopy system consisting of a control and acquisition unit, the display and control interface, and the laser illumination and detection unit (*A*). Microscopic images are generated in vivo using the handheld confocal microscopy probe by direct placement onto the tumor-tissue to be evaluated (*B*). After tumor induction by SSTR-positive rat pancreatic tumor cells (AR42-J) in nude mice, SSTR-positive tumor cells were selectively visualized after OcF application using the miniaturized CLM-system (*C*). After 30 minutes, a subset of tumor cells displayed a homogeneous cytoplasmatic staining pattern. SSTR-distribution was irregular among tumor cells and showed excellent correlation to ex vivo immunohistochemical staining of AR42-J tumor cells (anti-SSTR2-DAB) (*D*).

in 7 patients with biochemical evidence of pancreatic NET, both DOPA-PET and CT failed to detect the tumor.[41] In a recent prospective single-center study by Koopmans and colleagues[23,42] of 53 patients with metastatic carcinoids, both the region-based and lesion-based sensitivity was higher for DOPA-PET than for SSTR scintigraphy and for the combination of SSTR scintigraphy and CT. In pancreatic endocrine tumors, the sensitivity of DOPA-PET was slightly lower.

However, studies using somatostatin-receptor PET instead of somatostatin-receptor scintigraphy could not confirm superiority of DOPA-PET versus SSTR imaging. In the study of Putzer and colleagues[43] when comparing ^{68}Ga-DOTA(0)-Phe(1)-Tyr(3)-octreotid (DOTATOC)-PET and DOPA-PET, each modality showed a sensitivity of 64% and a specificity of 100% on a patient basis. Both imaging modalities showed equal findings in 7 of 15 patients and disagreement in 8 patients. DOTATOC-PET revealed more metastases than DOPA-PET in 6 patients, whereas DOPA-PET detected more metastases in 4 patients. However, overall, 208 malignant lesions have been detected by DOTATOC-PET, whereas only 86 lesions were found by DOPA-PET. In another series of 25 patients with GEP-NET, ^{68}Ga-DOTATATE-PET proved to be clearly superior to DOPA-PET for detection and staging of NET. DOTATATE-PET delineated 54 of 55 positive metastatic tumor regions compared with only 29 with DOPA-PET.[44] In conclusion, these studies demonstrate that when PET tracers are used for somatostatin-receptor imaging, DOPA-PET does not show an overall higher sensitivity for the detection of NET. Because SSTR imaging does not only offer diagnostic information but can be decisive for further treatment management, such as peptide-radioreceptor therapy, in patients with GEP-NET, SSTR-PET should be used as the initial functional imaging method. However, in patients with NET with negative SSTR imaging, DOPA-PET should be considered as a valuable second-line alternative.

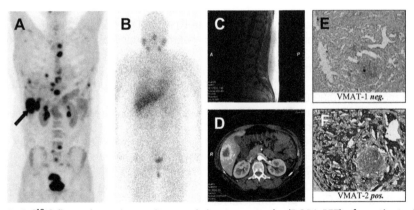

Fig. 5. 6- [18F]-fluorodopamine positron emission tomography (DOPA-PET) of a patient with metastatic retroperitoneal paraganglioma (A). In contrast to DOPA-PET imaging, none of the lesions had been detected with I-123-MIBG-scintigraphy (B). DOPA-PET shows metastatic lesions in the spine and in the liver, as well as paragangliomas in the head and neck area (the DOPA-PET–positive lesion in the right lobe of the liver adjacent to the large liver metastasis corresponds to a normal tracer uptake by the gall bladder; arrow). Corresponding to the lesions found with DOPA-PET, MRI (C) of the spine shows multiple hypointense tumors in the thoracic and lumbar spine. CT (D) of the abdomen reveals 3 hypervascularized liver metastases. Immunohistochemical analysis of the tumor demonstrated a lack of VMAT-1 expression (E), which predicts MIBG negativity, in contrast to a strong expression of VMAT-2 (F).

18F-Fluorodeoxyglucose-PET

Whereas ^{18}F-fluorodeoxyglucose-PET (FDG-PET) depicting glucose metabolism is generally an excellent tracer for a variety of tumors, highly differentiated neuroendocrine tumors may be FDG-PET negative. When comparing FDG-PET/CT with DOTA-TATE-PET/CT in pulmonary neuroendocrine tumors, DOTATATE-PET/CT showed higher and more selective uptake for all typical carcinoids, whereas in atypical carcinoids with a higher proliferation index, FDG-PET/CT sometimes showed higher uptake.[45] In another study for typical pulmonary carcinoids, a mean SUV of only 3.0 was found.[46] In line with association of FDG-PET uptake with lower tumor differentiation, FDG-PET is a strong prognostic marker.[47] Therefore, in addition to SSRT imaging, FDG-PET might play a role in detecting biological properties on a lesion-by-lesion basis in a concept of individualized therapy (see **Figs. 2–5**).

Alternative Radiotracers for Positron Emission Tomography

As a PET-tracer analogue to MIBG, ^{11}C-hydroxyephedrine (HED) has been established, mainly for imaging of cardiac adrenergic innervation.[48] In a comparative study, HED PET could detect more overall lesions than MIBG-SPECT in patients with neuroendocrine tumors (80 vs 75).[49] Depicting similar pathways than [18]FDOPA, the tracer ^{11}C-5-Hydroxy-L-Tryptophan has been applied in clinical studies. However, because of the similarity with [18]FDOPA and the shorter half-life of ^{11}C, its application is limited. Other peptides like [111]Indium-minigastrin, targeting the pentagastrin-binding receptor (CCK_2), or radiolabeled exendin-4, targeting the glucagonlike peptide 1 receptor, have been proposed for peptide imaging.[15] In another recent study, gastrin-receptor scintigraphy provided additional information as compared with SSTR scintigraphy in selected patients with neuroendocrine tumors.[50]

REFERENCES

1. Ploeckinger U, Kloeppel G, Wiedenmann B, et al. The German NET-registry: an audit on the diagnosis and therapy of neuroendocrine tumors. Neuroendocrinology 2009;90(4):349–63.
2. Klimstra DS, Modlin IR, Coppola D, et al. The pathologic classification of neuroendocrine tumors: a review of nomenclature, grading, and staging systems. Pancreas 2010;39(6):707–12.
3. Modlin IM, Oberg K, Chung DC, et al. Gastroenteropancreatic neuroendocrine tumours. Lancet Oncol 2008;9(1):61–72.
4. Oberg KE, Reubi JC, Kwekkeboom DJ, et al. Role of somatostatins in gastroenteropancreatic neuroendocrine tumor development and therapy. Gastroenterology 2010;139(3):742–53.
5. Eriksson B. New drugs in neuroendocrine tumors: rising of new therapeutic philosophies? Curr Opin Oncol 2010;22(4):381–6.
6. Cimitan M, Buonadonna A, Cannizzaro R, et al. Somatostatin receptor scintigraphy versus chromogranin a assay in the management of patients with neuroendocrine tumors of different types: clinical role. Ann Oncol 2003;14(7):1135–41.
7. Krenning EP, Kwekkeboom DJ, Bakker WH, et al. Somatostatin receptor scintigraphy with [111In-DTPA-D-Phe1]- and [123I-Tyr3]-octreotide: the Rotterdam experience with more than 1000 patients. Eur J Nucl Med 1993;20(8):716–31.
8. Kowalski J, Henze M, Schuhmacher J, et al. Evaluation of positron emission tomography imaging using [68Ga]-DOTA-D Phe(1)-Tyr(3)-Octreotide in comparison to [111In]-DTPAOC SPECT. First results in patients with neuroendocrine tumors. Mol Imaging Biol 2003;5(1):42–8.

9. Gabriel M, Decristoforo C, Kendler D, et al. 68Ga-DOTA-Tyr3-octreotide PET in neuroendocrine tumors: comparison with somatostatin receptor scintigraphy and CT. J Nucl Med 2007;48(4):508–18.

10. Shankar LK, Hoffman JM, Bacharach S, et al. Consensus recommendations for the use of 18F-FDG PET as an indicator of therapeutic response in patients in national cancer institute trials. J Nucl Med 2006;47(6):1059–66.

11. Nikolaou A, Thomas D, Kampanellou C, et al. The value of 11C-5-hydroxy-trypto-phan (5HTP) positron emission tomography (PET) in neuroendocrine tumour diag-nosis and management: experience from one center. J Endocrinol Invest 2010. [Epub ahead of print]. PMID: 20332708.

12. Fottner C, Helisch A, Anlauf M, et al. 6-18F-fluoro-L-dihydroxyphenylalanine posi-tron emission tomography is superior to 123I-metaiodobenzyl-guanidine scintig-raphy in the detection of extraadrenal and hereditary pheochromocytomas and paragangliomas: correlation with vesicular monoamine transporter expression. J Clin Endocrinol Metab 2010;95(6):2800–10.

13. Christ E, Wild D, Forrer F, et al. Glucagon-like peptide-1 receptor imaging for localization of insulinomas. J Clin Endocrinol Metab 2009;94(11):4398–405.

14. Mansi R, Wang X, Forrer F, et al. Evaluation of a 1,4,7,10-tetraazacyclododecane-1,4,7,10-tetraacetic acid-conjugated bombesin-based radioantagonist for the labeling with single-photon emission computed tomography, positron emission tomography, and therapeutic radionuclides. Clin Cancer Res 2009;15(16):5240–9.

15. Reubi JC, Maecke HR. Peptide-based probes for cancer imaging. J Nucl Med 2008;49(11):1735–8.

16. Zhang H, Chen J, Waldherr C, et al. Synthesis and evaluation of bombesin deriv-atives on the basis of pan-bombesin peptides labeled with indium-111, lutetium-177, and yttrium-90 for targeting bombesin receptor-expressing tumors. Cancer Res 2004;64(18):6707–15.

17. Brogsitter C, Pinkert J, Bredow J, et al. Enhanced tumor uptake in neuroendo-crine tumors after intraarterial application of 131I-MIBG. J Nucl Med 2005; 46(12):2112–6.

18. Kratochwil C, Giesel FL, Lopez-Benitez R, et al. Intraindividual comparison of selec-tive arterial versus venous 68Ga-DOTATOC PET/CT in patients with gastroentero-pancreatic neuroendocrine tumors. Clin Cancer Res 2010;16(10):2899–905.

19. Reubi JC, Schar JC, Waser B, et al. Affinity profiles for human somatostatin receptor subtypes SST1-SST5 of somatostatin radiotracers selected for scinti-graphic and radiotherapeutic use. Eur J Nucl Med 2000;27(3):273–82.

20. Kwekkeboom DJ, Krenning EP. Somatostatin receptor scintigraphy in patients with carcinoid tumors. World J Surg 1996;20(2):157–61.

21. de Herder WW, Kwekkeboom DJ, Valkema R, et al. Neuroendocrine tumors and somatostatin: imaging techniques. J Endocrinol Invest 2005;28(Suppl Interna-tional 11):132–6.

22. Kwekkeboom DJ, Krenning EP, Scheidhauer K, et al. ENETS consensus guide-lines for the standards of care in neuroendocrine tumors: somatostatin receptor imaging with (111)In-pentetreotide. Neuroendocrinology 2009;90(2):184–9.

23. Koopmans KP, Neels OC, Kema IP, et al. Improved staging of patients with carci-noid and islet cell tumors with 18F-dihydroxy-phenyl-alanine and 11C-5-hydroxy-tryptophan positron emission tomography. J Clin Oncol 2008;26(9):1489–95.

24. Dromain C, de Baere T, Lumbroso J, et al. Detection of liver metastases from endo-crine tumors: a prospective comparison of somatostatin receptor scintigraphy, computed tomography, and magnetic resonance imaging. J Clin Oncol 2005; 23(1):70–8.

25. Gibril F, Reynolds JC, Chen CC, et al. Specificity of somatostatin receptor scintigraphy: a prospective study and effects of false-positive localizations on management in patients with gastrinomas. J Nucl Med 1999;40(4):539–53.

26. Zhernosekov KP, Filosofov DV, Baum RP, et al. Processing of generator-produced 68Ga for medical application. J Nucl Med 2007;48(10):1741–8.

27. Schottelius M, Poethko T, Herz M, et al. First (18)F-labeled tracer suitable for routine clinical imaging of sst receptor-expressing tumors using positron emission tomography. Clin Cancer Res 2004;10(11):3593–606.

28. Miederer M, Seidl S, Buck A, et al. Correlation of immunohistopathological expression of somatostatin receptor 2 with standardised uptake values in 68Ga-DOTATOC PET/CT. Eur J Nucl Med Mol Imaging 2009;36(1):48–52.

29. Gabriel M, Oberauer A, Dobrozemsky G, et al. 68Ga-DOTA-Tyr3-octreotide PET for assessing response to somatostatin-receptor-mediated radionuclide therapy. J Nucl Med 2009;50(9):1427–34.

30. Baum RP, Prasad V, Hommann M, et al. Receptor PET/CT imaging of neuroendocrine tumors. Recent Results Cancer Res 2008;170:225–42.

31. Goetz M, Kiesslich R. Advances of endomicroscopy for gastrointestinal physiology and diseases. Am J Physiol Gastrointest Liver Physiol 2010;298(6):G797–806.

32. Goetz M, Fottner C, Schirrmacher E, et al. In-vivo confocal real-time mini-microscopy in animal models of human inflammatory and neoplastic diseases. Endoscopy 2007;39(4):350–6.

33. Kiesslich R, Goetz M, Neurath MF. Confocal laser endomicroscopy for gastrointestinal diseases. Gastrointest Endosc Clin N Am 2008;18(3):451–66, viii.

34. Fottner C, Mettler E, Goetz M, et al. In vivo molecular imaging of somatostatin receptors in pancreatic islet cells and neuroendocrine tumors by miniaturized confocal laser-scanning fluorescence microscopy. Endocrinology 2010;151(5):2179–88.

35. Rufini V, Calcagni ML, Baum RP. Imaging of neuroendocrine tumors. Semin Nucl Med 2006;36(3):228–47.

36. Bombardieri E, Coliva A, Maccauro M, et al. Imaging of neuroendocrine tumours with gamma-emitting radiopharmaceuticals. Q J Nucl Med Mol Imaging 2010;54(1):3–15.

37. Havekes B, King K, Lai EW, et al. New imaging approaches to phaeochromocytomas and paragangliomas. Clin Endocrinol (Oxf) 2010;72(2):137–45.

38. Ilias L, Sahdev A, Reznek RH, et al. The optimal imaging of adrenal tumours: a comparison of different methods. Endocr Relat Cancer. 2007;14(3):587–99.

39. Ilias I, Chen CC, Carrasquillo JA, et al. Comparison of 6-18F-fluorodopamine PET with 123I-metaiodobenzylguanidine and 111in-pentetreotide scintigraphy in localization of nonmetastatic and metastatic pheochromocytoma. J Nucl Med 2008;49(10):1613–9.

40. Hoegerle S, Altehoefer C, Ghanem N, et al. Whole-body 18F DOPA PET for detection of gastrointestinal carcinoid tumors. Radiology 2001;220(2):373–80.

41. Ahlstrom H, Eriksson B, Bergstrom M, et al. Pancreatic neuroendocrine tumors: diagnosis with PET. Radiology 1995;195(2):333–7.

42. Koopmans KP, de Vries EG, Kema IP, et al. Staging of carcinoid tumours with 18F-DOPA PET: a prospective, diagnostic accuracy study. Lancet Oncol 2006;7(9):728–34.

43. Putzer D, Gabriel M, Kendler D, et al. Comparison of (68)Ga-DOTA-Tyr(3)-octreotide and (18)F-fluoro-L-dihydroxyphenylalanine positron emission tomography in neuroendocrine tumor patients. Q J Nucl Med Mol Imaging 2010;54(1):68–75.

44. Haug A, Auernhammer CJ, Wangler B, et al. Intraindividual comparison of 68Ga-DOTA-TATE and 18F-DOPA PET in patients with well-differentiated metastatic neuroendocrine tumours. Eur J Nucl Med Mol Imaging 2009;36(5):765–70.
45. Kayani I, Conry BG, Groves AM, et al. A comparison of 68Ga-DOTATATE and 18F-FDG PET/CT in pulmonary neuroendocrine tumors. J Nucl Med 2009; 50(12):1927–32.
46. Kruger S, Buck AK, Blumstein NM, et al. Use of integrated FDG PET/CT imaging in pulmonary carcinoid tumours. J Intern Med 2006;260(6):545–50.
47. Binderup T, Knigge U, Loft A, et al. 18F-fluorodeoxyglucose positron emission tomography predicts survival of patients with neuroendocrine tumors. Clin Cancer Res 2010;16(3):978–85.
48. Matsunari I, Aoki H, Nomura Y, et al. Iodine-123 metaiodobenzylguanidine imaging and carbon-11 hydroxyephedrine positron emission tomography compared in patients with left ventricular dysfunction. Circ Cardiovasc Imaging 2010;3(5):595–603.
49. Franzius C, Hermann K, Weckesser M, et al. Whole-body PET/CT with 11C-meta-hydroxyephedrine in tumors of the sympathetic nervous system: feasibility study and comparison with 123I-MIBG SPECT/CT. J Nucl Med 2006;47(10):1635–42.
50. Gotthardt M, Behe MP, Grass J, et al. Added value of gastrin receptor scintigraphy in comparison to somatostatin receptor scintigraphy in patients with carcinoids and other neuroendocrine tumours. Endocr Relat Cancer 2006;13(4): 1203–11.

Index

Note: Page numbers of article titles are in **boldface** type.

Gastroenterol Clin N Am 39 (2010) 937–945
doi:10.1016/S0889-8553(10)00107-X
0889-8553/10/$ – see front matter © 2010 Elsevier Inc. All rights reserved.

gastro.theclinics.com

United States Postal Service

Statement of Ownership, Management, and Circulation
(All Periodicals Publications Except Requestor Publications)

1. Publication Title	2. Publication Number	3. Filing Date
Gastroenterology Clinics of North America	0 0 0 - 2 7 9	9/15/10

4. Issue Frequency	5. Number of Issues Published Annually	6. Annual Subscription Price
Mar, Jun, Sep, Dec	4	$264.00

7. Complete Mailing Address of Known Office of Publication (Not printer) (Street, city, county, state, and ZIP+4®)

Elsevier Inc.
360 Park Avenue South
New York, NY 10010-1710

Contact Person
Stephen Bushing

Telephone (Include area code)
215-239-3688

8. Complete Mailing Address of Headquarters or General Business Office of Publisher (Not printer)

Elsevier Inc., 360 Park Avenue South, New York, NY 10010-1710

9. Full Names and Complete Mailing Addresses of Publisher, Editor, and Managing Editor (Do not leave blank)

Publisher (Name and complete mailing address)

Kim Murphy, Elsevier, Inc., 1600 John F. Kennedy Blvd. Suite 1800, Philadelphia, PA 19103-2899

Editor (Name and complete mailing address)

Kerry Holland, Elsevier, Inc., 1600 John F. Kennedy Blvd. Suite 1800, Philadelphia, PA 19103-2899

Managing Editor (Name and complete mailing address)

Catherine Bewick, Elsevier, Inc., 1600 John F. Kennedy Blvd. Suite 1800, Philadelphia, PA 19103-2899

10. Owner (Do not leave blank. If the publication is owned by a corporation, give the name and address of the corporation immediately followed by the names and addresses of all stockholders owning or holding 1 percent or more of the total amount of stock. If not owned by a corporation, give the names and addresses of the individual owners. If owned by a partnership or other unincorporated firm, give its name and address as well as those of each individual owner. If the publication is published by a nonprofit organization, give its name and address.)

Full Name	Complete Mailing Address
Wholly owned subsidiary of	4520 East-West Highway
Reed/Elsevier, US holdings	Bethesda, MD 20814

11. Known Bondholders, Mortgagees, and Other Security Holders Owning or Holding 1 Percent or More of Total Amount of Bonds, Mortgages, or Other Securities. If none, check box. ☐ None

Full Name	Complete Mailing Address
N/A	

12. Tax Status (For completion by nonprofit organizations authorized to mail at nonprofit rates) (Check one)
The purpose, function, and nonprofit status of this organization and the exempt status for federal income tax purposes:
☐ Has Not Changed During Preceding 12 Months
☐ Has Changed During Preceding 12 Months (Publisher must submit explanation of change with this statement)

PS Form 3526, September 2007 (Page 1 of 3 (Instructions Page 3)) PSN 7530-01-000-9931 PRIVACY NOTICE: See our Privacy policy in www.usps.com

13. Publication Title		14. Issue Date for Circulation Data Below
Gastroenterology Clinics of North America		June 2010

15. Extent and Nature of Circulation			Average No. Copies Each Issue During Preceding 12 Months	No. Copies of Single Issue Published Nearest to Filing Date
a. Total Number of Copies (Net press run)			1794	1600
b. Paid Circulation (By Mail and Outside the Mail)	(1)	Mailed Outside-County Paid Subscriptions Stated on PS Form 3541. (Include paid distribution above nominal rate, advertiser's proof copies, and exchange copies)	676	579
	(2)	Mailed In-County Paid Subscriptions Stated on PS Form 3541 (Include paid distribution above nominal rate, advertiser's proof copies, and exchange copies)		
	(3)	Paid Distribution Outside the Mails Including Sales Through Dealers and Carriers, Street Vendors, Counter Sales, and Other Paid Distribution Outside USPS®	495	441
	(4)	Paid Distribution by Other Classes Mailed Through the USPS (e.g. First-Class Mail®)		
c. Total Paid Distribution (Sum of 15b (1), (2), (3), and (4))	▲		1171	1020
d. Free or Nominal Rate Distribution (By Mail and Outside the Mail)	(1)	Free or Nominal Rate Outside-County Copies Included on PS Form 3541	124	106
	(2)	Free or Nominal Rate In-County Copies Included on PS Form 3541		
	(3)	Free or Nominal Rate Copies Mailed at Other Classes Through the USPS (e.g. First-Class Mail)		
	(4)	Free or Nominal Rate Distribution Outside the Mail (Carriers or other means)		
e. Total Free or Nominal Rate Distribution (Sum of 15d (1), (2), (3) and (4))	▲		124	106
f. Total Distribution (Sum of 15c and 15e)	▲		1295	1126
g. Copies not Distributed (See instructions to publishers #4 (page #3))	▲		499	474
h. Total (Sum of 15f and g)			1794	1600
i. Percent Paid (15c divided by 15f times 100)	▲		90.42%	90.59%

16. Publication of Statement of Ownership

If the publication is a general publication, publication of this statement is required. Will be printed
in the December 2010 issue of this publication. ☐ Publication not required

17. Signature and Title of Editor, Publisher, Business Manager, or Owner

[signature]
Stephen R. Bushing – Fulfillment/Inventory Specialist

Date
September 15, 2010

I certify that all information furnished on this form is true and complete. I understand that anyone who furnishes false or misleading information on this form or who omits material or information requested on the form may be subject to criminal sanctions (including fines and imprisonment) and/or civil sanctions (including civil penalties).

PS Form 3526, September 2007 (Page 2 of 3)

Moving?

Make sure your subscription moves with you!

To notify us of your new address, find your **Clinics Account Number** (located on your mailing label above your name), and contact customer service at:

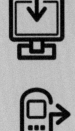

Email: journalscustomerservice-usa@elsevier.com

800-654-2452 (subscribers in the U.S. & Canada)
314-447-8871 (subscribers outside of the U.S. & Canada)

Fax number: 314-447-8029

Elsevier Health Sciences Division
Subscription Customer Service
3251 Riverport Lane
Maryland Heights, MO 63043

*To ensure uninterrupted delivery of your subscription, please notify us at least 4 weeks in advance of move.

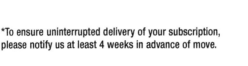